D0408986

YOU CAN DROP IT!

HOW I DROPPED 100 POUNDS ENJOYING CARBS, COCKTAILS & CHOCOLATE—AND YOU CAN TOO!

ILANA MUHLSTEIN, M.S., R.D.N.

This book is intended as a general reference volume only, not as any form
of medical treatment or advice. The information given here is designed
to help you make informed decisions about your health and wellness.
It is not provided or intended as any form of a medical diagnosis or plan,
or a substitute for any treatment that may have been prescribed by your doctor.
If you have any unique medical issues or conditions, or otherwise
suspect that you may have a medical issue or sensitivity,
please first consult with a medical provider before starting this or
any other nutrition program to discuss your specific needs.

You Can Drop It! Copyright © 2020 by Beachbody LLC.
All rights reserved. Printed in the United States of America.
No part of this publication may be reproduced or transmitted in any form or
by any means, electronic or mechanical, including photocopying,
recording, or any other information storage and retrieval system,
except in the case of brief quotations embodies in critical articles and reviews,
without the written permission of the publisher.

Design by Galvanized Media

Library of Congress Cataloging-in-Publication Data

Name: Muhlstein, Ilana, author.

YOU CAN DROP IT!
How I Dropped 100 Pounds Enjoying Carbs, Cocktails & Chocolate—And You Can Too!
Ilana Muhlstein

New York, NY
ISBN-13: 978-1-940358-46-8

Published by Beachbody LLC

www.beachbody.com

Distributed to the book trade by Galvanized Media and Simon & Schuster

To my mom, of blessed memory,
who always supported my transformation,
yet made me feel beautiful at every weight and size

CONTENTS

FOREWORD

By LISA LILLIEN, AKA HUNGRY GIRL

F YOU LIKE to eat, this book is great for you. And that means a lot coming from *me*—because my nickname is Hungry Girl and food is my passion! I've pretty much devoted my life to helping others make better eating choices—scouring shelves for smart swaps and sharing them with the masses in my daily emails, Hungry Girl books, magazine, podcast and on social media.

My followers live happier and healthier lives following my tips, tricks and recipes, which help them survive any and every eating situation, even in the hungriest of times. I hear from them a lot, and if there's one thing I've learned, it's that weight loss is nearly impossible to achieve if you don't have the right motivation. That's why I'm so grateful you're holding *You Can Drop It!*

My friend Ilana Muhlstein, M.S, R.D.N., will help you take off weight and *keep* it off thanks to a mindset that's proven to work. She has personally helped thousands of men and women lose 10, 20, 30, even 100+ pounds on her plan, the 2B Mindset. She's living proof that it works, having lost 100 pounds herself using the same techniques. *And she looks amazing!*

In *You Can Drop It!*, she shares the secrets of how her methods can change your body, and your life, revealing the physical and mental benefits that come with rethinking your relationship with food. And her Core Four principles are so easy to remember: Water First, Veggies Most, Use the Scale, and Track Your Progress. They're always there for you—every time!

Ilana's results are super impressive. And so is she! It's funny how much we have in common. We're both opinionated women from New York, and not afraid to be loud and proud. We both grew up overweight—her obese, me a little chubby. Our moms were both yo-yo dieters. In our homes as kids, food was not just for sustenance or pleasure; it was a topic of conversation, always. We lived through the weight-loss crazes of the '80s and '90s, for better or worse: grapefruit-only diets, cabbage soup diets, the Beverly Hills Diet (eat only fruit for 10 days). I remember thinking as a kid, "If you're on a diet, you're eating nothing that's bad for you. If you're off a diet, you can eat everything all the time." It was all or nothing. Black or white.

Years later, I realized that is not the way to live life and definitely not the best way to achieve your weight goals. That's when everything changed for me. I launched Hungry Girl in 2004 to help people make smart food choices and give them real-world eating solutions, strategies and easy recipes. To me, there's nothing more fun than getting in the kitchen (like a mad scientist!) and recreating something—replicating flavors by swapping out ingredients that are not so good for us with healthier ones. And of course, making everything taste delicious! I've been called a "foodologist," not because I have a fancy degree, but because I'm super into enjoying and appreciating food.

What I love about Ilana is that, in addition to her impressive degrees (plural!), she's a typical woman facing the same food issues most of us deal with every day, just like me. In *You Can Drop It!*, she'll be brutally honest about the struggles she went through when she was obese, what she learned in her years of study, and how she maintains her incredible weight loss today. The 2B Mindset is rooted in the soundest of nutritional intelligence, but it also comes from a place of truth.

After reading it, you'll be more honest with yourself, and this is a good thing. Ilana knows you're going to want that cinnamon bun. She knows you'll want to go crazy at that wedding buffet. She knows you might feel shame. And she makes that all okay with a plan that untangles your emotions about food and makes you feel clear, calm and cool about eating. This thinking has helped her private clients, and those who've signed up for the 2B Mindset online, be who they've always wanted to be. Now it's your turn. So grab your fork and dive in!

Enjoy the journey, and as I always say... Chew the right thing!

LISA LILLIEN
Founder, Hungry-Girl.com

INTRODUCTION

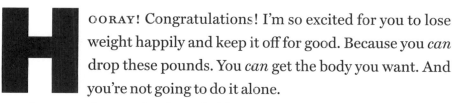

Welcome to the 2B Mindset!
You *Can* Lose Weight Without Feeling Deprived or Hungry Ever Again.

OORAY! Congratulations! I'm so excited for you to lose weight happily and keep it off for good. Because you *can* drop these pounds. You *can* get the body you want. And you're not going to do it alone.

There are thousands of people like you, unhappy in their bodies and wanting to change. I see them professionally, as a registered dietitian nutritionist with my own private practice. More than 240,000 others have signed up for 2B Mindset, my online course and system for simple and sustainable weight loss. These folks have shed 20, 30, 50, even 100+ pounds and rediscovered their best selves thanks to the unique, easy and effective guiding principles found within the program videos and resources—and in this book.

I know you can drop the weight because I dropped the weight—a *lot* of weight—using this very same plan. People say they can't believe it when they see me, but I grew up morbidly obese, weighing more than 200 pounds at my heaviest. I've been through this struggle. I know *exactly* how it feels. I get that there are temptations and cravings. I understand that big wins are usually followed by bigger setbacks. I know what it's like to feel like the body you're in doesn't reflect the *you* inside.

I also know that I lost 100 pounds—and that I've kept it off. I know that I still love food and eating lots of it. I know that I'm happier and healthier than ever before. And I know you can be, too. The techniques in *You Can Drop It!* work. They work because they're the result of proven methods combined with science-backed nutrition advice.

My clients pay more than $400 an hour for this counsel. After seeing how amazing they look and feel during our sessions together—and even months and years later—I knew I couldn't hold these solutions back from those who really need it. My lifelong goal is to help real people like you and me lose weight in the most empowering and enjoyable way possible. It thrills me to share my secrets with you here and even more at 2BMindset.com, because I am committed to have this work for you.

Inside you'll get practical strategies to help you learn how to eat with purpose, live your life and lose weight so you can keep it off for good. And although I'll motivate you along the way, I'm not just some rah-rah cheerleader (though if you say I look like one, I won't complain!). I am a Registered Dietitian Nutritionist (the highest standard in nutrition). I have a Master of Science in nutrition. I sit on the prestigious Executive Leadership Team for the American Heart

Association and lecture for the Bruin Health Improvement Program at UCLA. I'm in the National Weight Control Registry—that's the longest study out there on weight loss in America of people who lost weight and kept it off. And I created the 2B Mindset with Beachbody, the pros behind P90x, INSANITY, and other fitness programs that have helped millions of people get the bodies they deserve from the comfort of their homes.

I also have a degree in tough love or PYF—pushing you further. I might seem too direct at times, but I believe hard work equals bigger results, and I am obsessed with results, namely yours. You only get one body, I always say. So you might as well make it rock!

To join in, you don't have to buy into some new fad or spend thousands on exercise equipment or give up carbs forever. You just need the right guidance and a new...mindset.

GETTING INTO THE 2B MINDSET

This is probably not the first time you've attempted to lose weight. I'm sure in the past, you've gained some weight and—maybe after being inspired or embarrassed or frustrated—decided it was time to lose it. What did you do? Maybe promise yourself you would fast or cleanse or try really, really hard to eat perfectly for a day, a week, or a month. And maybe you even succeeded. And I give you credit for your willpower, because I never stood a chance using those methods.

Or maybe all of that strictness, discipline and effort frustrated you because you only saw a little success and felt like a failure. So you got sluggish and sad. Your energy crashed, and you went looking for something to make you feel better. Why, hello, leftover cookies and jar of peanut butter!

2B MINDSET SUCCESS STORY

Brandi S., an Independent Team Beachbody Coach, 36, Lake Charles, Louisiana, lost 106 pounds in 15 months*

"You found a way that made eating healthy and losing so simple!"

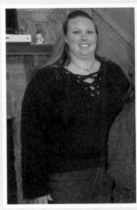 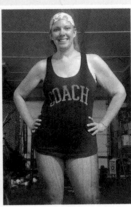

*Results vary depending on starting point and effort and following Beachbody fitness programs.

MOST PEOPLE HAVE an unhealthy idea about weight loss—that it involves making sacrifices, emotionally obsessing over food and, overall, enjoying it less—but it doesn't have to be that way. This is one of the things that many of my clients realize after spending just a few weeks on the 2B Mindset program. Brandi was 274 pounds on day one of the program, and in a little over a year dropped more than 106 pounds—while forging her best-ever relationship with food. "You found a way that made eating healthy and losing so simple!" she tells me. "There were simple instructions"—Water First, Veggies Most, Use the Scale, Track Your Progress—"but I was still able to have all my favorite things."

The biggest benefit of 2B Mindset for Brandi wasn't the weight she lost, but the sense of self she has gained in the process. "The 2B Mindset has helped my self-confidence so much," she says. "It completely changed my outlook every day and with interactions with others. I still have struggles with emotional eating, but now I know how to properly cope!"

That's when you gave in—and felt guilty that you did. So you chose to wave the white flag and surrender... again.

And your weight went back up... again.

That mindset doesn't work—and it hasn't worked for millions of people struggling with their weight who have been trying those same methods.

The mindset that does work—as shown by hundreds and hundreds of my clients and the hundreds of thousands more who have used this program—is the 2B Mindset. Why? Because the 2B Mindset is designed to be sustainable from day one. It doesn't shame you for your love of food, busy schedule, skipped workouts, or lack of meal prep; it works with you and your real life! It redefines your relationship with food and with how you think about eating. You won't ever be told to cut out sweets, but the cool thing is, once you have a new mindset, you may never want them the same way. And it starts with having a good relationship with your body, which, as a result, also leads to super-effective weight loss.

Ultimately, the 2B Mindset is rooted in this fundamental truth about nutrition: Weight loss is about what food you eat, but it's also about your eating behaviors, reaction to hunger and food environments, and how you can figure out what works best for you and your body.

We all have different bodies, we all like different foods and we all have different lifestyles and schedules. For you to have long-term success—and a healthy relationship with food and your body—you have to understand that successful weight loss isn't about rigid meal plans and deprivation. A way of eating has to be about what's in your mind as well as what's on your plate.

Life throws you curveballs, and the 2B Mindset equips you with the tools you need to smash them—not the other way around. This program is designed to help you handle any struggle or hurdle you face because it's not about being "perfect," but about being customized.

Here's what you stand to gain.

Freedom

The 2B Mindset is not a diet. You're not going to count calories, you're not going to calculate grams, you're not going to cut out food groups, you're not going to permanently swear off alcohol, sweets or anything. The second you start telling yourself "no," you're just going to be stuck on that, and that's the last thing you want. Are you skeptical or wondering how and why that's possible? Despite what you read, do you still think you should cut out bread to lose your weight? Let's try this little exercise and see if it works for you.

Try not to think about elephants. Whatever you do, for the next minute, don't think about elephants. Don't think about their grayish color, the way they walk, their floppy ears or long trunks.

How'd you do?

See, not that promising.

With the 2B Mindset, you're going to be telling yourself "yes." You'll focus on the positive and what works for you, and all you need to start is an open mind.

Control

One of the things that I hear most often from people who have the 2B Mindset is something I enjoy even more than hearing that people lost weight. They report that they finally have control. There's so much in life that feels out of our control. And in many cases for women, what happens to their bodies is out of their control (puberty, PMS, pregnancy, nursing, menopause, etc....sorry if that's TMI, boys, but it's the uncomfortable truth for us). Our bodies are constantly morphing away from us, and we just want to get control of our weight, shape and abilities. I know how this feels, and I know so many others who feel the same, too. Getting control of your mindset and eating habits allows you to finally get control of your body—and your interactions with and emotions toward food.

Short-Term, Long-Term and Sustained Weight Loss

Everything that comes from the 2B Mindset revolves around my Core Four—these four principles that will give you the weight loss, the freedom and the control you want: Water First, Veggies Most, Use the Scale, and Track Your Progress. No intense food rules, calorie counting, strict meal plan regimens, drill-sergeant directives of must-do-this and gotta-do-that. The groundwork is based on these four highly proven and effective core principles—principles that will guide you and shape you to get the body that you want so you can feel better and live better.

When you put all that together, you'll find that the 2B Mindset is a health and weight-loss gift that keeps on giving. It makes life easier. It makes life fresher. It makes you brighter. It makes you more energetic. It's better for your joints; it's better for your back. It's just *better*. Weight loss is what's yummy, satisfying and delicious. But don't worry, you'll still be indulging in delicious food as well.

Throughout the book and program, you will get thousands of tips, tricks, strategies and pieces of information that can and will help you.

Weight Loss by the Numbers

WANTED TO MAKE sure the 2B Mindset truly worked for every type of person with every kind of lifestyle. At Beachbody, we enrolled 42 participants to test the program over the course of about one year. (Since goals varied for participants, the length of their participation varied between three and a half months to a little over one year.) Their results were absolutely incredible, and I am so proud of them for letting go of their old mindsets, creating new healthy habits and forming a positive relationship with food once and for all!

- Collectively the group *lost 1,743.4 pounds*!
  That's almost 9 baby Asian elephants!

- As a group, they *lost 1,451.2 inches*.
  That's the length of about 7 adult elephants!

- Fourteen participants lost between 10 and 30 lbs.

- Seventeen participants lost between 31 and 50 lbs.

- Eleven participants lost between 51 and 94 lbs.

- Everyone lost at least 5 percent of their body weight.

- And they reported having a better relationship with food overall.

What you won't find is a prescribed list of meals and when to eat them. I don't believe in that. If someone told me to eat asparagus and chicken for dinner one night, and then my husband told me he wants to get sushi, I'm going to want to get sushi with him, *but* also make it work for my goals. So there's no prescribed "thing." Forget the old mindset, where eating vegan/keto/paleo/macro/fasting/counting points is required for obtaining and sustaining your goals. The 2B Mindset is eating with a sensible yet flexible approach that is needed for physical and mental health.

Once you figure out your own system, the weight drops off, off, off. And it becomes second nature. What makes this different from other diets is that we are doing this together. I live with the 2B Mindset every day. I may be in "Maintenance Mode" (which you'll read more about on page 275) but I always have to be conscious. I laugh when I see people look me up and down and size me up as a "naturally thin" woman who seems too carefree to have ever struggled with her weight. No one understands how hard I had to work to get to where I am (unless they know me personally, of course). I still watch my weight. Every. Single. Day. More so than ever, because I'm not just living for myself and right now. I'm living for my future. I'm living for my husband, Noah, our daughter, Olivia, our son, Julian, and the whole 2B Mindset community.

As a result, no one wants this plan to work for you more than me. Everything I will push you to do is for the benefit of you because I care about you! You'll get to the weight you want to be. You'll forget the stories of the past. You're going to let go of this identity of someone who struggles with their weight, and you'll get to that place where you always wanted to be—to that person who is strong, fit and free.

So let's leave the past behind us and turn the page to focus on everything you want 2B.

xoxo,

Ilana Muhlstein, MS. RD.N.

THE 2B MINDSET AT-A-GLANCE!

I've made the 2B Mindset as simple as possible. The 2B stands for my "two bunnies," because when you make a peace sign with your two hands—one finger for each of my Core Four principles—it looks like you're making two bunny ears. True story: I came up with the name when I had just had Olivia, and I was reading her a nursery book that had two bunnies on it. But it also stands for What Do You Want 2B? Who Do You Want 2B? Now get to Where You Want 2B!

WATER FIRST

- Water helps keep you full so that you can make better food choices throughout the day.

- You should drink half your weight in ounces at a minimum each day. Your weight in pounds _____ ÷ 2 = _____ daily minimum goal in fluid ounces. For example, 180 pounds ÷ 2 = 90 ounces, which is just three 2B Mindset water bottles!*

- Try to drink 16 fluid ounces/480 milliliters before each meal (even before your morning cup of Joe!).

- You'll soon see that the more water you drink, the more weight you may lose.

---

* To calculate milliliters, multiply the fluid ounces by 30, so 16 fl. oz. x 30 = 480 ml.

VEGGIES MOST

- Veggies make you feel full and satisfied (and keep you healthy), so eat lots and lots of them throughout the day.

- The more meals that include "Veggies Most," the more weight you can lose.

- Find veggies you love and make them your go-tos. But also explore some you've never tried before—because you never know what you may like!

- Veggies can be enjoyed in hundreds of ways. Check out my recipes later in this book. There are also dozens more of our delicious recipes and recipe videos online within the 2B Mindset and The Mindset Membership.

THE SCALE

■ The scale is your friend! I know you may hate it or have been told to avoid it, but you'll soon see that it helps you learn what helps your body lose weight and what doesn't.

■ Get on the scale every morning, without clothes, after using the bathroom, before you eat or drink anything.

■ If you don't have a scale, get one and put it on a flat, hard surface, where you can easily hop on it every day.

■ When the scale goes down, you'll discover what a "weight-loss day" looks like. And should it go up or stay the same...you'll learn what to change to get right back into weight-loss mode.

TRACKING

■ Tracking is incredibly important. Your tracker will show you what's working for you and what's not.

■ Every day, complete a "My Day" page in your tracker book (which you can get at 2BMindset Tracker.com).

■ You decide how detailed you want to be, but the more details you put in, the more insights you will get out. Whatever you do, be honest— because this is for your benefit.

■ It will take your guesswork, guilt and confusion out of eating and boost your weight loss and maintenance success.

■ It only takes a few minutes each day. So, if you bite it, write it; if you drink it, ink it; and if you nibble it, scribble it.

These Core Four simple guiding principles are sensible and—best of all— sustainable, so you'll not only know how to lose the weight, you'll discover how to keep it off.

MOTIVATION STARTS RIGHT HERE

I Dropped 100 Pounds and You'll Drop the Weight, Too.

OUR LITTLE WORDS. After a decade of studying nutrition and working with private clients, I've discovered the number one reason why people can't lose weight, and it comes down to four little words. No, it's not "Pass me the pie" or "Make that a double" or even "Domino's, it's me, Ilana."

No, the four little words are: "I can't lose weight." I've never met anyone who has said with conviction, "I can't lose weight," and then lost weight. Think about it. It doesn't happen.

That's why I've developed a plan that centers around resetting your mindset. You will start thinking: "I *can* lose weight." In fact, you will see that your body loves losing weight! I know you may be rolling your eyes in disbelief and may want to slam the book down right now. I get it. I've taught weight loss seminars at UCLA for many years and used to ask the class to repeat after me, "I can lose weight," "I will lose weight," "I care to lose this weight," and "My body loves losing weight." I would lose some people at the first one but most by the fourth one. I know you may think that you have a metabolism slower than molasses in January. Believe me, I do too. But although you may think that you can't lose weight, you need to remember how badly your knees, joints, heart, back and organs want you to get leaner and healthier. Plus, you wouldn't be reading this book if you didn't think you had something of a chance, so you may as well take on the "I can drop it" mindset, because you can actually do this!

JUST TWO POUNDS AT A TIME

F YOU'RE SKEPTICAL, that is totally fine, and expected.

The main causes for doubting your ability to lose weight and keep it off I've identified are:

- You feel like you are so far from your goal.

- You haven't been able to lose weight and keep it off long term in the past.

- You feel like your current circumstances make it impossible for you to be successful.

My answer to that is:

- You're going to be able to reach whatever healthy and realistic goal you set for yourself, but the more you focus on that big number, the worse your motivation will be. You need to focus on losing *just two pounds at a time*. I truly and sincerely lost my 100 pounds by focusing on losing just two at a time. It will make you more determined, disciplined, hopeful and happy every step of the way. Whatever weight you are now, subtract two pounds for your first goal. You will get there (very likely this week).

- You've never lost weight with me—and this book—before, so don't make assumptions based on the unsustainable attempts in your past. Be open to writing a new story for your future because this time, this way, it's more than possible for you to succeed. I made a strong promise to myself many years ago that all weight loss and nutrition advice I share must be simple, sensible and sustainable. It makes all the difference, and you will see that for yourself.

- You will realize that no matter how difficult your circumstances, you can drop this weight. And by the end of this book (but hopefully sooner), you'll believe it, and even start to see it.

My clients—and the hundreds of thousands who've done the 2B Mindset online—believe it. The common ground between each of their success stories was a changed mindset that motivated them to redefine their habits to hit their goal weight. I have even heard from several dietitians and fellow health practitioners who watched my videos that although they heard similar insights before, I presented it in a new way that clicked in a new way. They had to forget what they'd heard or tried to follow in the past. They had to welcome weight loss and this new process so it could actually happen. They learned to believe their bodies *wanted* it to happen. Only then—armed with my easy and effective nutrition tips and strategies—were they able to break free of old habits, eat without sacrifice and keep the weight off.

Four words are all that's standing between you and the body, and life, you want.

In the coming chapters, you'll learn how to turn your old mindset into a new mindset, and discover the three pillars of weight loss, how to stop self-sabotage and more. You'll learn to cut the BS and unlock your greatest potential. But first, I want to get into the specifics of how motivation can lead to weight loss, and the real-life physical and mental benefits. I want to tell you how it worked for me—how changing my mindset saved my life.

Repeat Aloud

I mean it, with volume. I don't care who's around!

I CAN LOSE WEIGHT.

I WILL LOSE WEIGHT.

I CARE TO LOSE THIS WEIGHT.

MY BODY LOVES LOSING WEIGHT, AND SO DO I.

I CAN LOSE WEIGHT.

I WILL LOSE WEIGHT.

I CARE TO LOSE THIS WEIGHT.

MY BODY LOVES LOSING WEIGHT, AND SO DO I.

I CAN LOSE WEIGHT.

I WILL LOSE WEIGHT.

I CARE TO LOSE THIS WEIGHT.

MY BODY LOVES LOSING WEIGHT, AND SO DO I.

I CAN LOSE WEIGHT.

I WILL LOSE WEIGHT.

I CARE TO LOSE THIS WEIGHT.

MY BODY LOVES LOSING WEIGHT, AND SO DO I.

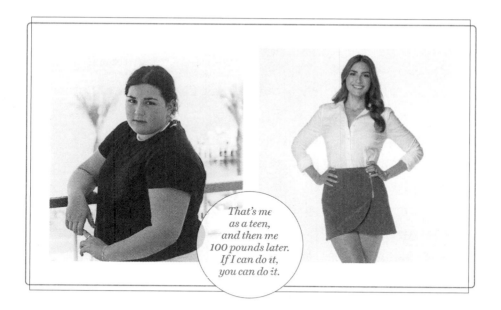

That's me as a teen, and then me 100 pounds later. If I can do it, you can do it.

I'M MORE THAN A PRETTY FACE

F YOU AND I met, you might think I was naturally lean, born with a fast metabolism, able to eat whatever I want without gaining a pound. Not gonna lie, that would be amazing. But the truth is, growing up, I was always the big kid. I was never "normal." I was never small. The pediatrician's office constantly told my parents, "She's obese. She's over the hundredth percentile—she's not even on the chart!"

I was about four years old when my parents got divorced, and every picture of me since then I was either trying to hide my body behind someone else or holding food. I guess I was using food as a form of comfort and a form of consistency when a lot of things in my life were inconsistent. Going to an amusement park, I'd immediately wonder: "What snacks are we packing? Ice cream cones!" "We're going to the circus? Cotton candy!" "We're going to a birthday party? Pizza! And cake!" As a kid, this is what I was thinking about. I turned to food for stability during those unstable times. Lots of take-out Chinese food, lots of sweets, lots of peanut butter—lots of *everything*.

I also didn't have the best role models. My family always struggled with weight and what to eat. My parents did every diet in the book, every fad—Atkins, South Beach, The Zone, Pritikin; today it'd be keto, paleo or detox juice cleanses. Just whatever was "in." I watched them try and struggle and gain it all back and more.

And I just kept getting bigger.

And bigger.

I saw the other girls in ballet chuckle about me behind my back, so I tore off my leotard and swore to never go back. I wasn't able to wedge into my friends' clothes on sleepovers. The pain of not fitting in hurt almost as much as "chub rub," the horrible chafing of my inner thighs. But the phrase that affected me more than any insult was: "You have such a pretty face." That I got told all the time, in a sad way. My grandparents, teachers, friends' moms: "You have such a pretty face." The implication being: "I'm a waste of space," or "Shame about the rest of you."

And it *was* a shame, for my health. According to my doctor, even as a teenage girl, I was experiencing blood sugar issues that "you would typically see in older men," she told me. I faced elevated blood pressure and cholesterol, and the potential for worse—and was at risk for diabetes or an early death. When I was just eight years old, my pediatrician looked my mom in the face and said, "You have to send her to a weight loss camp. She's going this summer."

So, at eight years old, I was shipped off to "Fat Camp." Can you imagine how that felt?

But the truth is, once I got over the sense of rejection from my family, I actually loved it. I made lots of friends. I was surrounded by people who didn't judge me. I lost 30 pounds after following their strict eating regimen, working out, and getting weighed and measured weekly. The good news was, at a very young age, I had a positive association with weight loss because I got so many compliments when I returned home.

I looked at this summer camp as something that was improving my life.

Then I came back to school...and gained it all back. This yo-yoing went on for years. Every summer, I'd lose 30 pounds. Every school year, I'd gain it all back—and more. I fell into a bad cycle. I became dependent on the two-month crash course to weight loss because I saw how easy it was for my body to gain weight (sometimes 45 pounds in less than 45 weeks!). But it's also likely that the deprivation was causing me to eat like crazy when I was "allowed." Perhaps it was just that I hadn't found the 2B Mindset yet, and no diets I tried ever worked. All I know is that I felt uncomfortable and large in public, I felt bad for enjoying food, I felt deprived of fashion and flirting and fitness and fun.

One year, I peaked. I had 215 pounds on my five-foot-two-inch frame, and was a size 20—and I was just 13 years old. A 13-year-old who was buying women's plus size clothes. I hated my body. It's sad to admit but I really did. I constantly fantasized about waking up to a new one and getting a fresh start, but it never came. It was all so unfair. I was filled with jealousy for skinny people. I had a horrible dependency on comfort food, diets and deprivation, all at the same time—and a really negative mindset.

Thankfully, something was different that summer going into high school, something that gave me extra motivation. I'd had enough. Suddenly, I really wanted not just to lose the weight but to keep it off. I had to break out of it. I always wanted to be trim, fit, healthy, strong and not to have my weight drag me down. So, that's when I just changed my mindset and I said, "Enough is enough." I got over the idealism that one day I would win the new body lottery and finally came to terms with the fact that it would only be possible if I put in the work. I asked myself, *"What did I do every summer that made it easy for me to lose weight? And what did I do differently during the school year that made it easy for me to gain the weight back?"*

At weight loss camp, even on a restricted diet, there were certain foods that I could eat as much as I wanted, and I'd still lose weight. I also knew that I liked to eat a lot of food. I was what you'd call a "volume eater"; I needed to feel full and satisfied. So I decided to try that on my own. I focused on the foods I could eat lots of, that made me feel satisfied, but that didn't cause me to gain weight. And by the end of my freshman year of high school, I was shocked. For the first time—all on my own—I'd not only managed to maintain my summer weight loss, I'd actually dropped even more pounds during the school year! On my own! For the first time ever in my life! I was so excited. I had discovered the formula that worked for me. It wasn't a new diet—it was a new *mindset*. It involved small and simple tweaks to my food environment, nutrition selection and emotional reactions, and it made all the difference.

Once I embraced it, I kept on losing weight, all through high school and when I went to college. Eventually, I got down to my first big goal of 145 pounds. Dietitians and doctors always showed me where I fell on the BMI charts, and at my current height of five feet, four inches, 145 pounds finally meant no longer obese or overweight, but just "normal and healthy." Finally, for the first time ever, I felt strong and confident. I was so happy at 145 pounds. I was "normal." My whole life my weight was my identity and a burden to myself and everyone around me and, finally, I was able to just be me. I was a size 8—the lowest size I'd been since I was eight years old. I was a single digit! And the best part was that I was able to maintain that weight, without denying myself or telling myself "no" all the time. You know what might be the most amazing part? It was a lot easier than I thought it would be. I always felt full and satisfied. I never deprived myself. And I never missed a meal. I just relied on a few simple principles—the ones in this very book—that allowed me to lose weight while still living my life. Because that's everyone's ultimate goal, right? To be happy. That's still

2B MINDSET SUCCESS STORY

Bethany J., 27, New York, New York, *lost 80 pounds in 20 months**

*"I needed a good kick in the a**."*

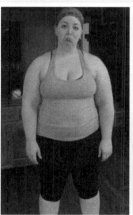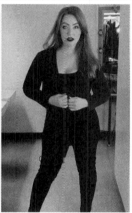

*Results vary depending on starting point and effort.

I LIKE TO SAY the best time to start 2B Mindset is anytime, but particularly when you're at rock bottom. Bethany J.'s been there. "I was the biggest I have ever been and feeling hopeless about it because I felt too far gone," she told me. She was willing to try anything, but she couldn't find a program that worked for her.

What finally made the difference was learning about important dietary tips and strategies—such as the ratios of how to "plate" each of her meals—that changed her mindset. In addition to losing over 42 pounds in three months, she says that the program gave her a new sense of optimism. "I feel lighter both physically and mentally," says Bethany.

A little tough love helped push her along, too. I don't sugarcoat anything, in my videos or one-on-ones. Says Bethany: "I needed a good kick in the a** and for someone to not accept my bullsh*t excuses." Her biggest piece of advice for anyone considering 2B Mindset is simply to do it. "Just commit regardless of what anyone around you says or any other 'educated information' you've read or heard," she suggests. "It works for everyone!"

my goal as a registered dietitian and nutritionist, wife and mom. And that's exactly why I wrote *You Can Drop It!*

SO MANY REASONS TO COMMIT

YOUR STORY IS different than mine. But we both have struggled with our weight and wished we didn't have to ever again. It was only after examining what it is we all have in common that I was able to develop a plan that works for everyone, a plan that's different from anything you've ever seen or tried.

You see, once I finally started to lose weight, I was determined to be a credible expert in nutrition. And I'm proud to say I did go on to get my bachelor of science degree in nutrition and dietetics, my registered dietitian license, and my master's degree in nutrition and dietetics because I wanted to make sure that I was advising people on the best and healthiest way to live, backed by scientific research. I can tell you which foods to eat so you'll never feel hungry again, and how to cook them, too—and in fact, later in this book, I will!

But it's funny because I actually speak less about nutrition than a lot of other health and wellness "gurus," because once I started going into practice, and started to counsel so many people, I realized, whoa, the nutrition approach is just a part of this. It's just one third. It's just one pillar.

Knowing what to eat is an important foundation. Understanding *why* you eat is equally essential. So the other pillars of weight loss, besides nutritional (as in, what we eat), are emotional (why and how we eat) and environmental (where, why and with whom we eat). In the next chapter, I'll get into why each can make or break your weight loss.

The genesis of this breakthrough was on the lips of every client who came to see me; we talked more about their struggles than about recipes for kale salad. "I'm going through this divorce and I can't stop eating cookies." "I lost a parent." "My boss is codependent and I have no room to breathe." "Life is short and I can't resist a good party." So what did they do? They ate. We emotionally eat when we're stressed, when we're happy, when we're excited, when we just feel like we're missing out on a good time. That's why I ate. That's sometimes why I *still* eat.

So I started developing more processes, more tools, more "Ilana-isms," more sayings, more *everything* to help you deal with the emotional and environmental factors that inform weight loss because I needed them for myself too! I saw that action begets action—while also of course delivering the best nutritional foundation. (Through the process, I also got married and had my first child, Olivia. Talk about an emotional and environmental change!)

That's when I met the team at Beachbody. At that point, I had thousands of clients. I'd lost a hundred pounds, had tons of testimonials to prove it and show it, and taught at UCLA (and continue to lecture there). Beachbody and I took my ideas one step further—5,000 steps further actually. We improved it, created more tools, more resources,

---

Ilana-ism

Positive People = Positive Weight Loss

The more positive your mindset, the more positive your weight loss. As you continue your progress, be sure to surround yourself with uplifting and supportive influences—including those whom you follow on social media and those with whom you spend your weekend. And if you ever feel like you don't have that kind of support, that's when you can lean on our incredible exclusive community when you join The Mindset Membership! You'll learn all about that later on.

tested the 2B Mindset on hundreds of people and continued to refine it. We served our first test group at the end of 2017. Three years later, people are now down 70, 80, 90, 95 pounds. We have two folks down 95 pounds and they have kept it off.

The Three Modes of 2B Mindset

As you adopt the 2B Mindset, you'll go on a journey from "kinda getting it" to "every day is a weight loss day."

WEIGHT LOSS MODE

In the early stages, you'll adopt new habits and a new mindset, and will be learning, losing and leaning on the program principles. Experiment with new recipes, foods and mealtimes. It takes trial and error, working through old habits and adopting new ones. You can get ongoing support from me through The Mindset Membership Exclusive Community. You can find all the info about the membership at the-mindsetmembership.com.

- *Expected duration: 3–6 weeks of full focus*
- *Expected weight loss 0.5–2.5 pounds a week.*

MELTING MODE

At this point, you no longer crave your old favorite foods because you've associated them with trigger foods that don't lead to weight loss results. You're now really into at least four to five different veggies or dishes and have never drunk so much water. (In fact, you wonder how you survived drinking so little before.) You're in love with the scale and realize now that avoiding it in the past was doing you no good. Tracking is second nature, and you know that "if you bite it, you should write it." You've seen your ability to lose weight even when treating yourself so you're not scared to be honest with it. Once it's clear what weight loss days look like for you, consistency is key. You now know how to effectively plan ahead for events physically (like bringing a veggie platter) and mentally (fending off food pushers).

- *Expected duration 2–60 weeks*
- *Expected weight loss: 1–3 pounds a week, every week. Until you hit . . .*

And it's all thanks to this positive framework, change of the mind, elevation in education and reshaping habits that didn't benefit them. Your mind is your steering wheel, and wherever you turn it, that's where you'll be. Once you turn it toward "I can do it"—which will

MAINTENANCE MODE

You got to your goal weight! Knew ya would. And you're going to have no problem staying there. You'll still be drinking Water First, and still be eating Veggies Most, because that's probably what you're used to eating anyway. These habits just remain habits, and they make you feel good—why stop them? You'll still be comfortable with the scale and keep loving it after it gives you that positive reassurance. And once you hit your goal weight you will continue to track, for at least six weeks, because you're already in the habit of writing down what you're eating. And it might just mean some extra room for cocktails or bites of treats on the weekends. Once you're super-clear on what Maintenance Mode looks like for you, you might be able to ease off the tracker a bit. Because while Water First, Veggies Most and the scale are all key components in weight loss and maintenance, the tracker is more a necessity of weight loss and laying the foundation for maintenance. However, know that you're never to be "above tracking," because in the future, once you've maintained your weight for a while you may encounter a slight weight gain due to a holiday, stressful time or vacation. Thankfully, staying consistent with the scale will help you take notice of a 5–10 pound-gain and be able to get back on track, rather than ever having to deal with a 20+ pound gain ever again. If this should happen, you will want to return to the tracker, because in just a few days, with muscle memory and discipline, you'll be able to get right back into that happy maintenance range.

■ *Expected weight loss: A lifetime—of happiness!*

strengthen your resolve to follow the Core Four—the benefits are endless. Here's what'll happen if your results are anything like those who followed my teachings.

You'll Lose Weight

Like, a lot! As I said, some folks have lost 100 to 150 pounds, and you'll meet some of them in this book. But just as Rome wasn't built in a day, it didn't take a day for you to eat the way you do. It'll take some time to change it. Don't be discouraged if you don't see a *ginormous* weight loss like you might if you'd done some deprivation diet or quick-fix— although you should still lose weight right away.

You'll End the Downward Spirals

The most effective time to start the 2B Mindset is when you are fed up with being fed up. I suspect this is because we're all more motivated to avoid pain than we are to seek pleasure. For instance, growing up, I dreamed of the benefits of being thin and wearing short skirts, but I never really thought it could be a reality, so I'd keep gaining weight. What drove me to change was fearing how painful it would be to continue to drag my weight struggle into the next stage and chapter of my life. Over the years, I've noticed my most successful clients have been motivated to avoid experiencing the same pain or illness as their parents or loved ones; fear of not being fit enough for their kids, spouse or grandkids; fear getting up to a certain size or number on the scale; or fear of how they will look and feel at a milestone event like a wedding. So, while you may really hate where you are starting out from, that may work to your advantage if it brings you a sense of urgency and propels you to work harder and stay more focused.

If you're feeling at the bottom of a downward spiral, know this isn't the end for you. It's the starting point for your future. Sometimes the

2B MINDSET SUCCESS STORY

Darlene D., an Independent Team Beachbody Coach, 38, New York, New York,
lost 84 pounds in 16 months*

"My confidence and self-esteem improved!"

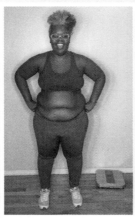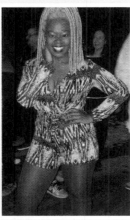

**Results vary depending on starting point and effort
and following Beachbody fitness programs.*

EXCESS WEIGHT CAN have a serious impact on your health—and also your identity. When Darlene D. was first introduced to 2B Mindset, she struggled to get up the stairs to her fourth-floor walk-up apartment.

"Physically, I had no energy," she confessed to me. "Every time I would get up the steps and into my apartment, I would have to sit down for a few minutes to catch my breath." It left her feeling completely lost, and she had surrendered to the harsh reality that she would be obese forever—even though she was only in her mid-thirties!

However, the program gave her a new lease on life—and she had lost more than 74 pounds in less than a year! "Once I decided that this just might be my last time to get my life right, I was on the correct path," she says. In addition to her changed mindset, she found my "Water First, Veggies Most" Ilana-ism particularly helpful. "It really isn't that difficult," she adds. "This way of eating is my norm now."

future feels much further away than you realize. But it's actually close. The time between now and then will come with change, momentary sacrifices and some difficulty—but you will come out the other side so much stronger, happier and more confident. You'll be faced with choices and points of discomfort as you steer away from your past. There's comfort in self-sabotage. But there is also very little that's comforting about where you are now.

You can bridge the gap between "I gained weight and am frustrated" and "I am motivated!" and can make the push to start losing weight and make changes now.

You'll Cut the BS

It's important to accept yourself at every size and strive to be a happy, confident person no matter what you weigh, but I'm guessing you don't really want to be overweight or obese. I certainly didn't! And you know what? That's okay! I know that may sound controversial. The #bodypositive movement—encouraging people to love their figures instead of shaming them—was born out of good intentions. But the problem is, it's led people into thinking it's one or the other: that you can either be body positive *or* you can lose weight. Choose both!

I've worked with several people who have told me they'd really want to lose weight, but their friends tell them that they shouldn't or don't have to. You might have friends that think it's okay that you've been gaining weight. Hey, they might say, you've got a busy career or a second kid or financial stress or a demanding relationship—why add a diet to your troubles? Love your body, love yourself, at every size, they say. And here, have more wine.

To me, that's not being such a good friend. In fact, I'd say to that person, "Here I am, trying to get healthier and more confident in my body, and do something good for me, and you're telling me not to? Why should I pretend to be comfortable, when I am not the healthiest, best self I can be?"

There is a fine line between self-kindness and self-sabotage. In these moments where you or someone else is telling you to skip your workout or grab another cookie, it may seem thoughtful, but it could also be deleterious to your future self, who won't remember the taste of that cookie.

The truth is, at the end of the day, you have to take care of yourself. Saying you're "body positive" and then eating a box of pasta because you "love yourself and it's okay" and then feeling horrible afterward with low energy, heartburn, regret and excess weight on your body isn't really being body positive. It's being in denial.

Excessive eating has been made into a socially acceptable vice but one out of three Americans is obese and according to the CDC, obesity puts you at risk for many of the leading causes of death, including heart disease, stroke, some types of cancer, respiratory diseases, diabetes, and kidney disease. (Heart disease kills more Americans than all cancers combined.) Then there are the medical complications that don't necessarily kill you, like female infertility, arthritis, gout, and depression.

You know I can relate to all this. When I was 215 pounds and wearing a size 20, I wasn't sad and mopey. I was confident. I was one of the more

Ilana-ism

Self-Discipline is the Highest Form of Self-Love.

We are faced with more than 200 eating decisions every day.
Don't settle for ones that don't serve you or lead to where you want to be.

Truth and Consequences

To truly understand how you feel about your body, make a list of the consequences of being—and staying—exactly where you are now. Here's an example:

I have no energy and no confidence. I'm ashamed in the bedroom. I am self-conscious at restaurants. I crop myself out of every picture, have no clothes to wear, my back is hurting. I'm sweating more, breathing heavier, just all-over negative. The me inside feels different than the me outside.

Now do yours, here or in a journal:

_____

_____

_____

_____

Reread what you wrote. What is the most uncomfortable aspect of where you are now? What do you want to work on with the 2B Mindset?

Now write a paragraph from a future you—the you six months from now. How does she or he feel?

_____

_____

_____

_____

Whatever you put there is possible if you come to this with an open mind. An open mind is a changeable mind.

popular girls in school. I had a lot of friends, I was sociable, I was upbeat. I "loved myself at every size" because I've *had* to love myself at every size. And while I always dreamed of being slimmer, I didn't actually start losing weight until I admitted to myself that I actually cared to. That's the key word you want to remember. You have to be okay caring, because it's in the moments of "whatever, I don't care" that bad choices happen. You have to know why it's important for you to do this. In truth, health and clothes were not enough to motivate me. I decided I finally had to drop my weight so I could be more authentic to who I am and was meant to be. I always had energy and personality, and I finally became fed up living in an outer body that I didn't feel was a proper reflection of the strength and vivaciousness that I carried within. I felt trapped in a body that I didn't feel proud of. I had to change my mindset, and I had to take on an approach that would actually work.

So love your body enough to want to take care of it, work with it and improve it, but don't settle. Keep focusing on those next two pounds at a time. Don't stop until you get the body you truly want, deserve and will feel proud of!

YOU'LL LOSE MORE THAN WEIGHT!

PEOPLE OF ALL shapes and sizes have done my program and seen results—even if weight loss wasn't their thing. When testing 2B Mindset, a lot of Beachbody Coaches tried the program—many of whom are fitness aficionados with no weight to lose. Some were already really disciplined, fit, trim and lean but needed to learn the program in order to help me teach it. So it was an eye-opener when they served as some of the most spectacular testimonials, saying that even though they didn't have any fat to burn, they didn't realize how negative their relationship with food and their body was, and that this program

My Top Eight Tips for Losing Weight

*In this book, you'll discover how to drop the weight big-time.
These are the foundations.*

■ *Wake up and get on the scale daily.* Don't avoid it if you think you were "bad" the night before—it will help you go back to being stronger sooner and can help make the missteps less frequent.

■ *Drink at least 16 ounces—that's 2 cups—of water right when you wake up and immediately following a workout.* These are the easiest times to drink a lot of water because your body craves it most. And 16 ounces is a little less than what the 2B Mindset water bottle holds. You can easily drink that! #waterfirst

■ *Exercise is optional*—but it can be very helpful for strengthening the mindset. Two options here:

   Option 1: *Work out!* I have seen dozens of people lose tons of weight without exercise, but there's something about the sense of physical accomplishment and empowerment following a workout that propels a greater sense of self-care throughout the day. What's more? It's very, very good for you, even if it's just a walk around the block. And don't make time an excuse. Beachbody on Demand literally has hundreds and hundreds of options you can do, 30 minutes or less, and as soon as you roll out of bed, right in your home.

   Option 2: *Can't work out?* Commit to a goal of not treating your body like a trash can. If you keep that mantra in your mind ("I won't treat my body like a trash can"), it can give you the same sense of physical empowerment, especially when you're making the choice to dispose leftover junk food or politely decline an offer to take home the extra fries.

■ *Eat two cups—think of it as two fistfuls—of veggies by two p.m.* It will drastically improve your sense of food control and eating behaviors in the afternoon and later at night. #veggiesmost

If you're not tasting or enjoying sugary or fatty foods, stop eating them. Yes, even if you are in the middle of that piece of banana bread right now. Collapse it in a napkin and chuck it. There is room for weight loss when you follow these steps and still have the occasional indulgence, but there is no wiggle room for eating sweets "just cuz." Drop the fork. Drop the justifications. And you'll drop the pounds.

Keep your hands, mouth and eyes busy and distracted. If you are at a social event or place with lots of foods and temptations, place yourself far from the food table. "In sight, in stomach"—so physically change what you see and how close you are to the food. If you can't move away, look up. (Pro tip: Want to keep your hands and mouth busy? Grab water, coffee, tea or zero-calorie beverages to keep in your hands and drink away. If you are getting hungry, find veggies first. Can't drink or eat? Bring gum or mints with you and suck on them discreetly.)

Write everything down post binges and after episodes of overeating. If you haven't officially started using the 2B Mindset Tracker or the Beachbody app, then at least write down everything you ate following a period of feeling out of control. You can use a pen and the back of a receipt or scrap paper. Even in Maintenance Mode, I still do this if I feel like I went overboard (and yes, most people, even people you wouldn't suspect, feel like they overeat sometimes). Benefits of writing this down include:

Recalling which parts were probably not even worth it.

Sometimes seeing that it wasn't nearly as bad as you thought.

Realizing that you're probably due for a veggie and lean protein as your next meal and that overeating may have occurred because of a lack of either or both of those things before the fact.

Awareness that these foods aren't good for you to have around. Think about the corrective measures to keep them out of sight, out of mind for the future. Also, it'll make the foods you ate less tempting because now you've created this uncomfortable yet enlightening association.

■ ***Set reasonable short- and long-term goals.*** I constantly see
that my clients who sync their weight loss goals with their future
plans—such as trips—lose more weight and stay more encouraged
than those who don't. You always want to have a sense of urgency
keeping you consistent and excited. For example, set a goal for
maybe eight pounds down from a month from now. Or 30 pounds
by four months from now. Think about many occasions and
events that mark these times as monumental. Remind yourself of
these goals by embedding them within your calendar. Write it in
the 2B Mindset Tracker, and on sticky notes to post at your desk,
in your closet, on your bathroom mirror or on the fridge as well.

has given them a far more positive view of their body, their health and the
way they are eating. Said these Team Beachbody Coaches:

■ *"It really helped me get in check with my binge eating, and the
hunger triggers I allowed to control me. I am able to identify real
hunger vs. the lies of hunger I told myself for years, and am now
eating to fuel my day."*
—ALLIE D., PERRYSBURG, OH, LOST 11 POUNDS IN 2 MONTHS*

■ *"The scale no longer defines me but is simply a tool to see how my
body reacts to the food I eat. And tracking has taught me to understand the ups and downs of weight gain."*
—COBY M., OREM, UT, LOST 21.1 POUNDS IN 4 MONTHS*

> ■ *"I like how Ilana encouraged people to take responsibility for their choices and not take excuses. I didn't want to weigh in every day and I did. Lots of lessons there."*
> —JUDI F., OCEANSIDE, CA, LOST 120.5 POUNDS IN 18 MONTHS*
>
> **Results vary based on starting point and effort and following Beachbody's exercise programs and Ilana's 2B Mindset program.*

It's something that I've always seen in my private practice because I've worked with so many people who just had disordered eating thinking, and I've worked with them to have a more positive mindset toward their health and their body.

Disordered eating is different than an eating disorder. Disordered eating describes a series of abnormal eating behaviors that, when considered alone, don't make up an eating disorder. For example, you may eat emotionally. Or you may eat compulsively. You may leave meals with feelings of guilt and regret. It's the conversation and negative self-talk surrounding the food that is the issue, rather than necessarily tied to a deeper mental or emotional disorder.

In the test groups, many Coaches said that they didn't realize that they would have a burger and fries, and then they would beat themselves up over it and compensate with excess exercise or deprivation. Or they had to do a super-hard workout the next day, because they would feel guilty about it, or they felt like they cheated. When you start doing 2B Mindset, you realize that isn't necessary. It's just a negative mindset. You're going to eat a burger and fries and say, "Okay, I had a burger, fries. It was delicious, but maybe I could have made some substitutions like ordered a side salad and tasted a few of my spouse's fries rather than had my own order. Now on with my day." It's that simple.

CHAPTER SUMMARY

■ *On 2B Mindset, you'll learn what to eat (and how to love the process), see that hard work pays off, end downward spirals and be more honest, leading to consistent weight loss.*

■ *Focus on losing just two pounds at a time. It will make you more determined and disciplined every step of the way.*

■ *Throughout the process, you'll implement the plan through trial and error (I call this Weight Loss Mode), master it and melt fat (Melting Mode) and then reach your goal weight and maintain it (Maintenance Mode).*

■ *I lost 100 pounds using these methods and am happier and healthier for doing so. This is the program for you if you have 5 pounds to lose—or a lot more. Others using 2B Mindset have dropped 100 to 150 pounds.*

■ *Never say or think these four dreaded words: "I can't lose weight."*

■ *Remember this mantra before starting and if the going gets tough: "I can lose weight. I will lose weight. I care to lose this weight. My body loves losing weight, and so do I."*

THE THREE PILLARS OF WEIGHT LOSS

Master the Nutritional, Emotional and Environmental Reasons You're Eating.

NEVER TRUST WEIGHT loss advice that hasn't been tested by the person giving it to you and proven to work *long term*! To test my ideas—and make sure that they worked on more people than just me—I had the most amazing "focus groups" imaginable.

It started when I graduated from the University of Maryland with a degree in nutrition and dietetics. By then, I'd learned the foundation of how to eat for better health, as well as for prevention and management of various disease states and medical conditions. I was simultaneously sharpening my own philosophies, tools and strategies that allowed me to lose weight while still living my life. (Yeah, I also partied and was in a sorority; don't hold that against me!)

I went on to a highly competitive program to become a registered dietitian nutritionist. It involved coursework, lectures and presenting research assignments through Cal Poly Pomona and City of Hope medical center, as well as ten months of supervised experience training to become a dietitian in clinical and community settings.

When I graduated, passed my board exam and earned my credentials, I was successfully down 75 pounds. UCLA hired me to counsel select staff members as part of a grant-funded program, and after a year of outstanding progress, in 2013, they basically said, "Ilana, here's a weight-loss seminar. We want you to lead it." So I took everything that I'd learned academically and through my own practical tips and advice and organized it into a 12-week course for which I enlisted 100 UCLA employees of every demographic. To be selected, participants had to apply for a lottery and have 40 or more pounds to lose. I had 19-year-olds working in the kitchen. I had 65-year-old secretaries. I had nurses working the late-night shifts, professors on their feet for most of the day, and dozens of people who sit most of the day in fund-raising, clerical, research and administrative-related jobs. We had women going through menopause, people with physical injuries who couldn't exercise and everyone in between. I started working out a system in that first semester that went relatively well. I only got to meet with the group once a week, and the average weight loss was about 10 pounds in 12 weeks, but I wanted to improve it. I kept teaching and tweaking the system from one semester to the next, while meeting with each person individually to get in the mindset of his or her relationship with food and to understand their lifestyle and goals. I went on to teach the course for ten semesters to a new group of diverse and interesting employees each time.

What Is the Right Weight for You?

Generally, you know your body—and your ideal weight—better than anyone, but there are times when it's important to check in with yourself a little. If several friends and family members are telling you to stop losing weight, there are a couple things you can do to double-check.

First, you can check your body mass index, or BMI. This is a simple calculation to help you verify that your weight is in a healthy range.

BMI CALCULATOR

To quickly calculate your Body Mass Index and learn if weight loss is appropriate for you:

BMI CATEGORIES*
Below 18 = Underweight
18.5-24.9 = Normal Weight
25.0-29.9 = Overweight
>30.0 = Obese

- *Multiply your weight, in pounds, by 703*
- *Divide that answer by your height in inches*
- *Divide that answer by your height, in inches again*

If your BMI is below the healthy range, talk to your health care professional. They'll be able to guide you in the right direction.

If, however, your BMI and health care provider confirm that you are in a healthy range and you feel like you are eating well, have good energy and are feeling physically strong and capable, be sure to silence those who may be interfering with your progress and stay the course.

Losing weight can be an amazing, life-affirming way to get the body that you've always wanted, and I'm so excited that you've decided to do it with me and the 2B Mindset community. Just keep these tips in mind to make 100 percent sure you stay your healthiest and feel most confident.

*"BMI Classification." Global Database on Body Mass Index. WHO. 2006.

As I kept perfecting the plan and structure, the weight-loss averages kept getting better and better—and better. The nutrition was a cornerstone, but I realized the difference was a mindset that was showing the greatest effect. Despite what I would assume on day one, sometimes the older woman going through menopause—the one you'd think have a harder time physically losing weight—would lose far more weight than a highly capable and active man in his twenties! I was in shock, and so was the class.

While building up my private practice, and working one on one with people, I noticed the same thing. I really started to understand where everyone was coming from and their weight-loss struggles—and how I could best help them overcome them so they could keep losing weight happily and learn to keep it off for good.

What I realized after years and hundreds of clients is this: All eating choices and behaviors are driven by one or a combination of the following three categories: Nutritional, Emotional and Environmental. These are the Three Pillars of Weight Loss that I am going to help you tackle.

Understand them and you'll understand why you eat the way you do, how you got to where you are—and how you're going to change it.

NUTRITIONAL

MOST DIET AND weight-loss books have relied solely on nutrition for weight-loss results. They'll have you cut out carbs, eat according to macros or points, drink only juice, eat low fat, eat like a caveman in the modern era (yet find yourself hunting and gathering your next slice of paleo-approved $18 pizza instead).

To illustrate why so many of these one-size-fits-all plans don't work in the long term, let's look at calorie counting as an example. Between the

2B MINDSET SUCCESS STORY

Matt H., 33, Brooklyn, New York, lost 40 pounds in 7 months*

"I had no idea that what I was eating was bad for me."

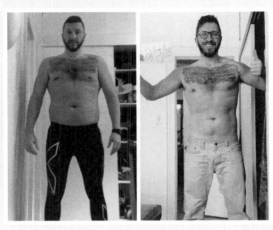

*Results vary depending on starting point and effort.

SO MANY PEOPLE I come across have a misunderstanding of health and wellness, which prevents them from achieving their goals. I rarely meet a new client who gained their weight from eating pizza and fries every day. It's usually someone in a frustrated state because he thinks he eats relatively well. Before Matt started the 2B Mindset, he thought he was living a healthy lifestyle. But despite the fact that he regularly went for runs and exercised, he could only maintain his weight—not lose any. "It was because what I was eating was actually bad for me, but I had no idea," he admits now.

Once he learned the 2B Mindset, he started making better food choices, sticking to foods that worked for him and "chugging water like it's nobody's business. I'm eating delicious food and loving it," he maintains. After his 40-pound weight loss he feels amazing—and also looks it. "I get compliments all the time," he admits. "That's really fun."

millions of downloads for the calorie-counting apps, and the restaurant menu calorie-count displays, it's a highly popular and widely attempted weight-loss method. People who say "calories in, calories out" try to attribute all of weight loss to this basic understanding of nutrition science. Yet it's clearly not that simple. Our society's struggle with weight and diets has only worsened as calorie counting has become easier.

The answer, simply put, is that different foods possess different abilities, and those abilities differ for everyone. Some foods are slower to be digested and may keep you satisfied longer—such as foods higher in fiber, protein and fat. Other foods break down rapidly, tricking you into eating more than you need—such as candy, cupcakes, juices and soda. Our gut microbiome and genetics also seem to dictate how we break down and store certain sugars, proteins and fats, and we're only just beginning to scratch the surface of that information. The point is that calories aren't created equal, and no single nutritional formula will work the same for everyone, or even for the same person in different stages of their life.

So while of course I am a dietitian with a master's degree in nutrition and have studied the breakdown of food to the nano level and will educate you in the importance of food in weight loss and health, I am going to present to you only the areas that you need and want to focus on. You will know what you want to eat, when and why, and will clear out the excessive, irrelevant and likely unsubstantiated advice that you've been given in the past.

(It's amazing how every influencer, friend and person standing next to you in the supermarket is a "nutrition expert" these days, isn't it? Well, despite what you've heard or seen in a documentary, there is no one perfect way of eating that works for everyone. You may have been told that you should go gluten free, dairy free, or become vegan, but why is it that those living in Ikaria, Greece—as written about in Dan

Buettner's *Blue Zones*—live eight years longer than Americans typically do, with half the rate of heart disease and almost no dementia, and follow none of these rules?)

The Core Four principles of the 2B Mindset—Water First, Veggies Most, Use the Scale, and Track Your Progress—are nutritional principles that really work. Every authority agrees that water and veggies should be the mainstay of our intake—and the scale and tracker help make this process your own. You are the best person to dictate what a perfect eating system looks like for you; when you begin to discover what food patterns bring you to your ideal weight and optimal health, you won't need to throw money and energy at a quick fix ever again. The Core Four principles make sense not just because they made sense for me when I lost 100 pounds, and not just for all my successful clients, both in private practice and at UCLA, but because they are also backed by research. What I love about the Core Four is that they're practical. There's no tallying numbers, cutting out whole food groups or messing up your social plans. No yo-yoing and jumping from diet to diet like it's a professional sport. (After seeing my parents go up and down on different diets, I vowed: "Wow, that definitely doesn't work, I never want to do that.") You will only focus on plain and simple nutrition that works.

And so, I found a way to make weight-loss food taste utterly delicious, but also something you will want to put in your body. And for that reason, *Girl Code* author Cara Alwill Leyba and hundreds of others have dubbed me the Food Hacker. (Because I've helped so many moms lose their baby weight, I've also been called the "MILF Maker," but that's a whole other thing.)

I could go on and on about my favorite foods. I truly don't discriminate. I love food. Always have and always will. No matter how much weight I had to lose or yearned to lose, I never sacrificed that level of enjoyment. But when you understand food as more than tasty but truly purposeful, it does help to change your cravings, habits and motivation.

Learning to choose the right food will also help you crave less of the food you don't want. You can truly eat more, lose weight and improve your self-control when you have a better understanding of nutrition and what to eat. So when crafting the nutritional guidelines for 2B Mindset, I knew the following had to be true:

The food has to taste good.

When I say eat "Veggies Most," I mean eat mostly vegetables, duh. What's unspoken is that you can top or mix those veggies with the toppings you love: melted cheese, sour cream, vinaigrettes, creamy dressings, toasted nuts and seeds, Thai peanut sauce, barbecue sauce, Everything But the Bagel seasoning and pesto. I promise no one ever gained excess weight eating salad dressing—you will see that food can and will be enjoyable, and how that will be a key factor in your adopting this as a lifestyle and maintaining this weight loss.

There has to be a lot of it.

As I said, I'm what you call a volume eater, but in fact most people are. Satiation and a sense of fullness are registered when there's a quantity of food present in our bodies. Don't feel ashamed for feeling deprived and hungry on other plans, failing. If you aren't full and satisfied, you'll never keep your weight off. There are no prescriptive serving sizes on the 2B Mindset. I like and need to eat a lot, and every day your appetite may be a bit different. In Chapter 7, I'll walk you through what and how I recommend eating to feel most satisfied.

There's no "cheating."

You can't cheat with 2B Mindset. You're only cheating yourself if you don't write it down. There's no one food or behavior that's forbidden.

Life will happen, treats, sweets and drinks will come up, and the key is to track them. I will walk you through the best way to go about dealing with them—what you want to have first, how to prioritize your favorites, and what to do if one serving has you wanting to go back for more—but you're not forbidden from experimenting, living and enjoying your life. And you'll see, you'll enjoy these things even more than you have before.

It has to be easy. Period.

Before long, you'll see that eating the 2B Mindset way is so easy—and even fun—that it seems like second nature. Sure, it will take effort in the beginning, but it will become effortless as you stay on it and with it. That's the bottom line when it comes to eating right. You shouldn't have to measure ounces of food or memorize a glycemic index. You just have to figure out what foods work for you *and* taste good to you!

What's Shakeology?

Throughout this book, you'll see me mention Shakeology, Beachbody's premier superfood nutrition shake. If you don't already drink it, that's fine, but you should know what it is and what it can do for you, because you might want to start. Shakeology was created to help you build a healthy diet foundation with its potent blend of protein, probiotics, fiber, digestive enzymes, adaptogens, antioxidants, superfoods, vitamins and minerals. Not only does it benefit your overall health, but the combination of protein and fiber can help you feel full and reduce your junk-food cravings—two important factors for anyone doing the 2B Mindset.

Every time I have Shakeology, I know I'm doing something amazing for my body and it's just going to set me up for a stronger day. If you want to learn more, go to teambeachbody.com.

EMOTIONAL

HAS ANYONE EVER said you're "big-boned"? Or that you have a "slow metabolism"? One doctor notified me I had "fat genes." I was told all that stuff my entire childhood. True or not, I didn't know, but they made for easy excuses. *I must be fat because I was born that way,* I'd think. And as the child of obese parents—whose own parents were obese—why would I think otherwise?

But eventually, I would start meeting friends and their families and say to myself, *You know what, they're actually eating differently than my family is.* They actually talk about food a lot differently than we do. My family: We were over-obsessed with food, and we were preoccupied with food. Food is all we think and talk about. It gives us anxiety and it gives us excitement and it's emotional and it's overwhelming.

I realized there is a more livable approach to eating well and living well. I realized it was about more of a mentality than a metabolism.

That's why I needed to start telling myself, and now I'm telling you, "You need emotional healing, not emotional eating."

If you're stressed, if you're sad, or even if you're just overwhelmed because you're hosting a party, or have people coming into town, or you have a huge to-do list and don't know where to start, sometimes you have to realize, "I need emotional healing. Not emotional eating."

We all need healing. Even if you're not going through a heavy time, you may need a break. A sense of relief. Life can be really hard. And when you start to identify what is overwhelming you and causing you to emotionally eat—pressure at work, budget concerns, politics, the death of a loved one, indecision, whatever it is—you can feel better by having more control over your eating.

Control brings calm. When I was a kid, we moved around a ton. I lived in eighteen different homes before I turned 20. My parents got remarried, they got divorced, they got remarried. I mean, we're talking a *lot* of instability, and food was always my comfort and my vice. I had one stool in the kitchen, right in front of the TV, and that was my safe place. No matter what food would come, I would eat, and eat, and eat. Jars of peanut butter, gifted desserts, dinner meant for the entire family that I would eat myself, leftovers, huge bags of rolls while walking home from school—I'd eat whole bags of rolls and be like, "What happened?" So I just kept getting bigger and bigger and bigger, as did my insecurities, which were fueling much of the process. It was a sad and toxic cycle of emotions and poor reactionary behavior.

Even today, I'm constantly re-introduced to my emotional eating self. But when you actually become real with it—and you realize the immense connection between your body and your choices—you also become very clear about what isn't working for you, which eventually becomes something you repel rather than crave. You also will discover new, healthy outlets for these feelings that you'll turn to soon as if they were second nature or muscle memory.

I wish everyone knew this, and I think we all do at some level. Emotional eating not only doesn't help us, it actually makes everything worse. When you're standing in your kitchen eating cold pizza or a carton of ice cream and thinking about your issues, your issues don't disappear when you reach the last bite. They're still there, and you know what you're left with? More issues than when you started. We all know that no matter the problem fueling the stress, food is unlikely to solve it. Unfortunately, however, our evil inclination of self-sabotage will momentarily suppress our better judgment and convince us that we don't care. I wish every person in the world would own their care. Of course you care. You wouldn't be reading this if you didn't. And it's a beautiful thing to care about your body and want to treat it properly. You only get one. It's the only thing no one can take from you; it's more valuable to you than the real estate in which you live! If you care about getting that cool new WiFi-enabled doorbell, or a foosball table for your rec room, but you don't care about your body, it makes no sense. None of that matters unless you believe *you* matter.

Yet so many of us pretend not to care. It's comforting to give up, because then you don't have to try. When you say you don't care, you give yourself permission to fail. This is especially true when those emotions lead, as they so often do, to weight gain. People gain weight for millions of reasons. I ask my clients, "What's your story? How'd you get to me?" And their answer is always long. A lot of times they think they're eating healthy but they make nutritional mistakes. A lot of times it's that they've moved in with new roommates who eat poorly. Sometimes it was sparked by an injury that caused them to stop working out. Or they got older and got a desk job. Or they never lost the weight postpartum, or gained weight following the death of a parent, or have a busy social life and traveling needs.

Running through each scenario, however, there is almost always an additional emotional piece, wherein their food relationship shifted from a place of purpose to a place of emotional comfort. I am a big fan of therapy and always encourage people to see and speak with someone. Some things are better addressed out loud with an unbiased professional armed with the tools to help you get to the bottom of these emotional voids, so you can improve mentally *and* physically.

I used to do this in my UCLA seminars and still do it with my private clients, and now it's your turn to try it, too. Say it out loud:

Emotional eating is never okay.

Again: Emotional eating is never okay.

While it seems silly now, you are actually embedding it into your subconscious and will be happy it pops up next time you need it. And while we're vocal and feeling amazing, let's try this one again:

> *I CAN LOSE WEIGHT.*
>
> *I WILL LOSE WEIGHT.*
>
> *I CARE TO LOSE THIS WEIGHT.*
>
> *MY BODY LOVES LOSING WEIGHT, AND SO DO I.*

SPECIAL SECTION

EMOTIONAL EATING A–Z

WHEN WHITNEY HOUSTON sang "I get so emotional, baby," I like to think she got the idea while eating Chinese food in her pajamas, alone on a stool in her kitchen at two a.m. I could come up with thousands of kinds of emotional eating, but here's a sampler. Which sound familiar to you?

- *Anger Eating:* When you're mad as hell and you're going to take it out on that poor bowl of egg noodles and butter or cereal and milk.

- *Avoidance Eating:* When you have a deep and latent issue, like the passing of a loved one or a dysfunctional relationship. You're eating rather than facing the deeper problem or insecurity.

- *Comfort Eating (of all kinds):* When you use food to soothe you, because you think you're too old for a pacifier. This can happen under any number of circumstances, including:

  On airplanes—You're a combination of exhausted, homesick and dehydrated and there's comfort in eating whatever the plane or hotel offers.

  PMS—Food is often not as much a biological need as it is a source of comfort when you may be feeling bloated and icky.

Under the weather—You would think people would lose weight when they're sick because they're either sleeping or filling up on tea and soup. Yet it's common for people to gain weight when sick. You're lying low and not exerting any energy. Friends bring you treats. You find comfort in a large matzo ball in your chicken noodle soup, in a large bagel or pasta.

■ ***Companion Eating:*** When eating together with a friend or spouse is what bonds you, and you continue to engage in unhelpful eating behaviors with this person (or people) because you fear there isn't a relationship without it.

■ ***Elevated Eating:*** When you don't eat from sadness as much as you eat from pleasure. For instance, if food was always a reward for you as a kid, this might stick with you as an adult. If every time you won a soccer game or got a good grade, you were treated to a restaurant meal and cookie, you may feel like every family or work celebration needs to be further enhanced by eating. While some people may be lonely and eat out of a longing for physical connection, others may eat to elevate their physical pleasures. I once had a client like this who lost his appetite when unhappy but became gluttonous when things were working well. He also created an association between making a snack and sex with his spouse, like a film noir antihero smoking a cigarette in an old movie (except with a sandwich).

■ ***Fear of the Unknown Eating:*** When you're unsure of an anticipated outcome, e.g., a high school senior waiting to hear back from colleges, or someone waiting for that all-important post-first-date text or a job applicant waiting for an offer—it can make a person mad, as in crazy. This can be a stronger feeling than even hate or anger. One may confuse this unsettling feeling in the stomach with hunger and suppress it with food for lack of a better option.

■ ***FOMO Eating:*** When you're in a group setting and feel as though you need to eat or drink with everyone else so you aren't left out. This happens frequently in the workplace when someone brings donuts. Another example is a bottomless brunch, where you feel you need to drink as much as your girlfriends to avoid their comments.

(P.S. Anyone shaming you for making a good choice for yourself is not a friend at all.)

- **Forced Eating:** When you feel obligated to eat something because someone else made it for you—made worse if they're guilting or pressuring you.

- **Guilty Eating:** When you fear getting thinner will make someone else feel bad. One of my toughest clients, early in my career, was a brilliant psychologist. She was so logically in tune with her self-sabotaging ways and knew precisely what she would have to do to lose the weight and keep it off. So what was the problem? One day she admitted to me that she can't slim down—for the sake of her sister. Her sister is still single while my client has a husband and kids. Her sister is lost in her career, and my client was the director of a department at a highly credible organization.

  Staying bigger, she felt, was a way of paying her sister back.

  Similarly, I've worked with mother-child duos in which the mom feels guilty if she loses more than the kid. Same has been true with couples. Sometimes the man loses a lot of weight while the wife struggles. At some point, either she is feeding him more or he feels guilty and creeps up to make her feel better.

- **Identity Eating:** When you were pinned as the big guy or girl or "eater of the family." That can be hard to break. I've worked with several people who weren't even big as a kid—just slightly bigger than their super-slim siblings—yet were still mocked. From then on they felt as though people were expecting them to eat. They felt as though they were "broader" by nature (even if they weren't at all!). This continued to haunt them late in their lives. See Chapter 9 for more about tools for changing your self-perception.

- **"Innocent" Eating:** When you say "one night of cookies" can't hurt, but you know full well that, for you, it leads to a downward spiral. A very innocent-seeming sweet woman I work with wants so badly to believe that "one night of eating fried bar foods isn't so bad," even though she sees how quickly it snowballs her into days and days of overeating, gaining weight and a feeling of *Ugh, I just don't want to* *eat anything healthy.* She does the same thing on Thanksgiving: "One night of pie can't hurt, it's the holidays." But by Sunday, she's finished the pumpkin, the apple *and* the mince.

Someone like this may also wish to be able to bake with her children and make cupcakes and cookies on a whim. The kids eat two. The mom eats 18 and then says things like, "I'm so mad at myself."

The saddest part of my job is sharing the reality of the person's tendencies. "You must know yourself, not test yourself." If you know that when you buy those chocolates "for the family," you end up eating them and get upset, then *stop buying them.* Same goes with baking. Kids don't need a mom who bakes; they need a mom with energy, confidence and good health. Kids don't need a perfect mom; they need a happy and, most importantly, healthy mom.

- *Lonely Eating:* When you're seeking companionship and want pleasure from a physical encounter.

- *Novelty Eating:* When you feel like you need to eat something because it's only available to you for a limited time like piña coladas on vacation or pie at Grandma's.

- *Procrasti-eating: My #1.* When you know you need to work to meet a deadline or run an essential errand but you justify needing to eat first. (Cigarette smokers do this, as well. Cigarette smokers do a lot of things on this list.)

- *Self-Sabotage Eating:* When you're well aware that you're doing something negative as you continue to eat. You may start to use justification and excuse language like, "It's okay, I'll start Monday" or "It's okay, I didn't eat all day or won't eat tomorrow." The example I use is that sometimes your phone falls and your screen cracks. You can either pick it up and get the screen repaired or take a hammer to it and demolish it. (When I used this example with a friend of mine who diets for sport, he said to me that I must not realize how fun it is to smash the phone. Ha!)

- *Silence Eating:* Rather than speaking up, you chow down. Everyone has a voice, judgments and observations. Extroverts are quick to share these thoughts. But others may be uncomfortable speaking up in public and may therefore resort to eating as a means of quieting themselves. Many of my larger clients are of the giving nature—so quick to care for and comfort and listen to others, and fearful of expressing their own needs and concerns. They feel guilty speaking up, asking for help and prioritizing themselves and may use food as their outlet to give back to themselves.

- **Spiritual Eating:** When eating is part of your religious custom. Judaism, for example, comes with a host of spiritually connected eating moments. For example, eating challah bread may be symbolic of good fortune. Eating honey on Rosh Hashanah symbolizes a sweet new year. When religion and spirituality are applied to foods, it adds a whole other layer of emotional eating.

- **Trash Can / Sense of Completion Eating:** When you don't want to waste food by throwing it away. If you grew up in a household that made you "clean your plate," you may relate. Often moms will eat off their kids' high chairs or you might be tempted to ask a friend at a restaurant, "Are you going to finish that?" It's important to tell yourself that "it's better in the trash than in my body" and "it's better in the waste than on your waist." Are you the type to keep eating because finishing it gives you a sense of accomplishment or completeness? For instance, you're done with the cookies but you would rather have the last one and be done with it than wrap it up or throw it away.

Y OU MIGHT BE an emotional eater and not even know it. A lot of people in our test groups claimed not to be emotional eaters. "I just didn't understand how to eat, and this program will help me do that." Then two months later they'll come back to me and say, " So I never *thought* I was an emotional eater, but my kid just went into the ER this weekend, and I found myself at the vending machine. Like, I had an emotional eating episode."

Well, yeah! We're *all* emotional eaters. There's no one person who is not an emotional eater. We are emotional beings and feel a host of emotions on any given day and also eat at three or more points a day. It's impossible for them not to collide. Anyone who says they're not an emotional eater just doesn't understand what that means. Happy, sad, angry, lonely, stressed, whatever it is—we're not robots, and those are emotions.

Food provides comfort. But caring about your body can provide a more lasting comfort. Weight loss gets easier when you go from, "I can't eat that" to "I don't want to because I am focused on my bigger goals." Here are a few ways to get there:

Identify why you're eating the way you are.

One thing that leads to big results is to ask yourself: "If I'm not hungry, why am I eating?" Are you eating the cake because you want to eat the cake? Is it a habit? Is it a form of comfort or self-sabotage even though you're not even tasting it? Is it because everyone else is eating? Is it because you have too much going on, and your life is really chaotic right now? That may not be something you can fix at the moment and that can be frustrating—but the cake is not going to solve anything. When you pause to ask yourself why and answer with "I'm just bored and feeling anxious," it can help you better understand your motivation.

Surrender yourself to something purposeful.

We all crave surrender. Life requires us to be so disciplined and attentive—in so many areas—that we all desire, at times, to throw our hands up, give in and veg out. It's human nature and it's okay, but it's important that you find a more purposeful form of surrender. Get a massage, treat yourself to new shoes, read a book or watch a show that's purely for entertainment, sleep in, say no to an invite or outing, get your nails done, plan a vacation or something else than feels indulgent and pleasurable yet not harmful.

Ease up on yourself.

Sometimes it is not others, but our own selves whom we are constantly disappointing. Reevaluate your standards and let go of judgment for yourself. Forgive yourself for the past. We all make mistakes, and we make them more often than we'd like, but we all deserve second (and third and fourth) chances. Treat yourself to forgiveness, and give yourself permission to move on from your past mistakes and take the opportunity to start over.

Mentor yourself.

I tell my private clients this all the time. You've got to mentor yourself because you're in your head all day. If you're eating something and saying that you're treating yourself, but the whole time you're thinking:

- *"This has so many calories."*
- *"Yeah, well, this is gluten-free."*
- *"I'm going to really regret this."*
- *"Is this even worth it?"*
- *"My kid is making me crazy."*

If at any time your head is getting distracted with:

- *"Oh, my God, I've got so many emails coming in."*
- *"I can't believe I have to go there later."*
- *"I'm so mad at him, I hate him."*
- *"She's such a b*tch."*
- *Or ... la la la...*

Whatever is going on in your head, if it's not "I'm fully enjoying this," if it's not, "This is delicious," I would say drop the fork—just drop the fork. The goal is to treat yourself, not cheat yourself.

Get productive, not destructive.

Oftentimes we eat as a form of reaction. I can't tell you how much of the weight in my client pool can fluctuate around an election. With every debate and political change comes a wave of stress eating after the nightly news. I get that the climate is tense right now and there is always something we wish to improve in our social, political and professional lives, but emotional eating is never okay. Repeat after me: "Emotional eating is never okay"—because it's destructive, not productive. What happens is, you're anxious and upset, so you start eating. Now you're more anxious, more upset—and guilty and regretful—than you were before. Stress eating increases your overall stress. When it comes to food and our bodies, we have to be more response-able, meaning more able to control our responses.

Instead: Get productive. Write a blog post. Read a book, watch a funny clip, drink a cup of tea, take a walk with your dog, hug someone or something, take a shower or bath, do something creative, call a friend, catch up with our Mindset Membership content. Do something that mitigates or alleviates your stress, puts you more at peace or resolve, and lets you rest up well. It's simple, but it's effective. Keep reminding yourself to be productive, not destructive.

ENVIRONMENTAL

WE ARE CREATURES of habit—you love potato chips in the afternoon, so you'll crave potato chips in the afternoon. We are also creatures of convenience—so you may love potato chips, but are you willing to drive to the 7-Eleven at eleven p.m. to restock if you're out? Probably not. If you want to lose weight, set up your environment so it's extremely inconvenient to gain weight, and extremely convenient to lose weight. The simple guideline is: "In sight, in stomach." So get your vices out of sight, and it will help to get them out of your mind and set of habits as well. At the same time, place everything in sight, in stomach that is serving you.

Your environment means people too, including your partner, your neighbors and your co-workers. I hear from my clients, "My spouse doesn't want to lose weight, and he keeps tempting me with things like ice cream and makes it harder." I'm sorry if that is the case, and I can relate 100 percent, so I need you to stand up for yourself and design your ideal weight-loss scenario, including the environment that's best for you and your relationships. Tell your friends and family what you're doing and call on them for their support.

I know you may roll your eyes, and you probably want to gloss over this point, but I need you to take the time to have these conversations. Healthy habits form healthy relationships. If your spouse eats his cookies in the kitchen before coming to hang out with you in the living room rather than tempting you with them on the couch, you will be so much more successful and thankful. On the other hand, if you allow everyone to tempt you and make it less likely for you to succeed, you may resent them as a result. I know this sounds harsh, but it can make or break your progress.

Your loved ones want to see you happy and succeeding, but you need to be clear with them how they can help you and don't assume they should just "know." When I was 25 pounds heavier and I first got married to my husband, we used to snack after dinner in the living room, which was right next to the kitchen. When I wanted to get serious and lose my last several pounds, I told him I wanted to relax in the bedroom after dinner and not in the living room, so I can get better at being "dinner and done."

My husband wasn't thrilled at first—but when he saw how proud, confident and grateful I was about accomplishing my goal, he was motivated to help support me. And if some nights I was tempted to stay in the living room with him—and fall prey to some handfuls of popcorn or leftover sweets—he would see how irritated I was by the setback and would feel bad.

I know it doesn't seem fair to ask others to adapt to our goals, but these are the people who benefit the most from us being our happiest, healthiest and most confident selves. Think about how much you do for them to make them happy and comfortable. They should be excited at the prospect of helping you, so let them.

Remember when I said "In sight, in stomach"? That also applies to food marketers and social media. Commercials for nuggets and fries at ten p.m., Pinterest recipes for ten-layer dip, and Instagram videos of chocolate lava cookies taking over your feed? Not really helping you! To overcome what I call "sense eating"—where you see it and you want to eat it—is to really look at who you're following on Instagram or on YouTube.

This goes for TV, too. Even as I was losing weight, I was obsessed with the Food Network. I have seen thousands of hours of the stuff. That's how I learned how to cook. Nowadays, if I check out the recipes flooding social media, and follow all these cakes and sweets, it's no surprise: it just makes me have sweet cravings and keep wanting to go back for sweets at night—food that I don't really want or need.

As individuals who are creatures of habit, what we see is what we crave and what we eat. This also applies to what we smell, touch, taste and even hear, whether that is the sound of popcorn popping or a *sssizzzling* steak getting cooked! Therefore, I always say:

For the perfect 2B Mindset fridge and pantry,
watch the **"Your 2B Mindset Kitchen"** video
online at 2BMindset.com.

Out of Sight, Out of Mind, aka OOSOOM

We have a lot of power when it comes to controlling the food that we consume daily. The more you put into practice the below points, the better control you'll have:

- Clear your kitchen countertop of the sliced bread, jars of cookies, leftover cake, soda and bowls of candy. If you think that they need to stay there for the other people who live with you, they don't. Just because they don't need to lose weight doesn't mean they should have these unnecessary things in their sight and stomach either. The entire household benefits by clearing it out.

- Replace those items with things to immediately quench hunger such as water, boxes of cherry tomatoes and bowls of fruit. Replace with bowls of apples, pears and tangerines, tomatoes, lemons, plants and winter squashes like spaghetti squash (they can last on your counter for up to three weeks!). When your kitchen is stocked with healthy, simple tools and ingredients, it can be easy to whip up delicious meals and actually want to eat them.

- Create other "stations" that encourage a healthy lifestyle, such as a tea or coffee station. You could also set up a Shakeology station with your favorite flavor of Shakeology next to a blender for a quick smoothie.

- Then clean out your car (toss the Big Gulp), desk and hiding spots (like your secret stash of Kit Kats in the top drawer in your nightstand).

- If traveling, you'll want to plan ahead. Ask the hotel to install a mini-fridge in your room—no, not one stocked with tiny bottles of tequila, but one you can stock yourself with your food.

Your 2B Mindset *Kitchen Guide*

When your kitchen is stocked with simple tools and ingredients it can be easy to whip up delicious meals. We've listed some go-to items you might consider keeping on hand.

Veggies

Meal Bases
(fresh & frozen)

Broccoli

Brussels sprouts

Cauliflower/cauliflower rice

Mushrooms

Onions

Pre-washed salad mixes

Slaw mixes

Spaghetti squash

Spinach

Stir-fry mixes

String beans

Zucchini

FFCs

Breads, whole-grain
(keep frozen, it lasts longer)

Frozen fruit
(great for smoothies)

Tortilla
(whole grain)

Waffles
(whole grain)

Whole fruit

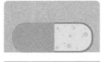

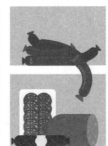
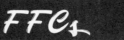

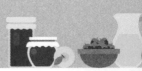
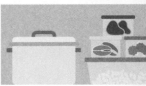
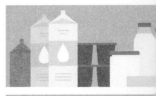
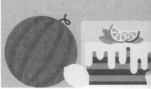
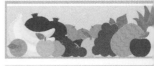
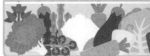

Fridge *& Freezer*

Veggies

Low-Maintenance, Grab 'n' Go

Baby carrots
Baby peppers
Broccoli florets
Cauliflower florets
Celery sticks
Cherry tomatoes
Cucumbers

Proteins

No-Cook, Grab 'n' Go

Cottage cheese
(1-2%)
Deli-cut slices, nitrite-free
(chicken, ham, roast beef, turkey, etc.)
Edamame
(organic)
Frozen pre-cooked shrimp
(defrosts in minutes!)
Greek yogurt
(plain, 0-2%)
Low-fat cheese
(cheese wedges, deli-cut slices, string cheese, etc.)
Pre-cooked grilled chicken or turkey
Ricotta cheese
(part skim)
Shrimp cocktail

Freebie *Accessories & Beverages*

Herbs
(fresh or frozen: basil, cilantro, dill, garlic, ginger, mint, parsley, etc.)
Hot sauce
Iced coffee
(unsweetened)
Iced tea
(unsweetened)
Lemon or lime juice
Low-sodium broth
(chicken, veggie, etc.)
Mustard
Salsa
Sparkling water
Water

Quick-Cook

Eggs/egg whites
Fresh or frozen fish fillets
(salmon, tilapia, tuna, etc.)
Fresh or frozen lean meats
(chicken, ground beef, turkey)
Frozen high-protein burgers
(chicken, lean ground beef, tuna, turkey, veggie, etc.)
Hard-boiled eggs
Tofu
(organic, extra-firm)

All Other Accessories

Almond milk
(unsweetened)
All-natural nut butters
(almond, peanut, etc.)
Full-fat cheese
(feta, goat cheese, etc.)
Guacamole
Marinades
Salad dressings
Shredded cheese
(keep frozen, lasts longer)
Soy sauce
(reduced sodium)

PANTRY

VEGGIES

Canned or jarred varieties of:

ARTICHOKES

BEETS

CARROTS

HEARTS OF PALM

PICKLES

SHAKEOLOGY BOOST: *POWER GREENS**

PROTEINS

BEACHBAR

CHICKEN

DAILY SUNSHINE*

SALMON

SHAKEOLOGY*

TUNA

FFCS

BRAN CEREAL (low-sugar)

BROWN RICE

CANNED BEANS
(black, chickpeas, kidney, pinto, etc.)

OATS

QUINOA

WHOLE-GRAIN CRACKERS

FREEBIE ACCESSORIES and BEVERAGES

ALL-NATURAL EXTRACTS

ALOE VERA

BEVERAGES AND WATER BOOSTERS

COFFEE, BLACK, UNSWEETENED

COOKING SPRAY

DRIED HERBS/SEASONING BLENDS
(garlic, onion, parsley, thyme, etc.)

DRIED SPICES
(cinnamon, cumin, paprika, pepper,
turmeric, etc.)

STEVIA (PACKETS OR LIQUIDS)

TEA, UNSWEETENED

VINEGARS, UNSWEETENED
(apple cider, balsamic
red wine, rice wine, white, etc.)

WATER ENHANCERS (all-natural flavors)

ALL OTHER ACCESSORIES

DRIED FRUIT
(cherries, cranberries, raisins, etc.)

MARINADES

NUTS, WHOLE AND CHOPPED

OILS
(avocado, grapeseed, olive,
toasted sesame, etc.)

POWDERED PEANUT BUTTER

SALT

SEEDS (chia, flax, etc.)

SHAKEOLOGY BOOST
*DIGESTIVE HEALTH, FOCUSED ENERGY**

*All products and flavors may not be available in your market.

KITCHEN

TOOLS

Recommended:

1 or 2 GOOD KNIVES

A FEW POTS AND PANS

CUTTING BOARD

BAKING SHEETS

MIXING BOWLS
(small and large)

VEGGIE PEELER

PARCHMENT PAPER
OR TINFOIL

PLASTIC WRAP

FOOD STORAGE BAGS

FOOD STORAGE CONTAINERS

OVEN MITTS

SHAKER CUP

SPATULA

Nice to have:

COMPLETE KNIFE SET

GRILL PAN

FULL COOKWARE SET

MANDOLINE

RUBBER SPATULAS

SLOW COOKER (CROCK POT)

FULL-SIZE BLENDER

FOOD PROCESSOR

SPIRALIZER

TONGS

2B MINDSET SUCCESS STORY

Jodi A., 39, New York, New York, lost 38 pounds in 7 months*

"If you put your mind to it, you can achieve anything you want!"

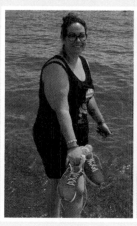 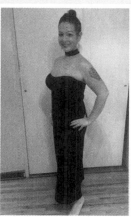

*Results vary depending on starting point and effort.

IT IS so beautiful to watch people's lives transform once they embrace the 2B Mindset approach, and Jodi is a prime example. Jodi really hit rock bottom when she was trying to get pregnant. Her doctor told her that part of the reason she hadn't yet been able to conceive was due to her weight and that unless she could lose weight, her chances of becoming a mother were slim.

She really connected with my story because we have similar backgrounds as overweight children. "I cried watching your video because that was me, my whole life," she told me. "I didn't feel alone, and you understood what I was going through."

Along with meal prep, one of the parts of the program that really helped Jodi was journaling, something she still does every day. "The most valuable lesson that I have learned from this program is that if you put your mind to it, you can achieve anything you want."

Ilana-ism

Dinner and Done, Find Other Fun

To avoid overindulging and overeating, get in the habit of being "dinner and done." You will have greater success if you plan to eat a more filling dinner, then plan on how you'll stop and find other activities to do.

CHAPTER SUMMARY

■ *The THREE PILLARS OF WEIGHT LOSS are:*
Nutritional (what you're eating),
Emotional (why you're eating) and
Environmental (the circumstances around which
you're eating). To break it down a bit more:

NUTRITIONAL: The Core Four principles of the 2B Mindset—Water First, Veggies Most, Use the Scale, and Write Down everything you're eating—are backed by research and really work.

EMOTIONAL: You need emotional healing, not emotional eating. There is a more livable approach to eating well and living well, and the secret is realizing it's more about mentality than metabolism.

ENVIRONMENTAL: You're in control of what you consume. Plan your kitchen accordingly, and keep things OOSOOM (Out of Sight, Out of Mind).

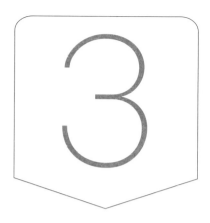

THE CORE FOUR

Meet the "2 Bunnies" That Lead to Weight Loss.

N 2B MINDSET, I will never tell you what you can't have. Our mindsets don't work that way. The second we're told we can't have something, that's all we think about, and all we do is think about how long we're going to be able to keep that up for and when we can retaliate. Instead of focusing on losing weight we become fixated on how we can't eat with our family, with our friends, at certain restaurants.

You feel isolated.

With 2B Mindset, you are always going to be focused on what you want to have, what you are eating and how much you're eating. Rather than thinking, *I can't eat that, I can't eat that,* you're going to be thinking, *I need more of that. I want more of that. I'm feeling so full. I'm feeling so satisfied.* It is so much more livable, effective and a positive approach to actually just eat well.

That's where my core four principles come in. No crazy things to remember, no hard calculations. What you're doing instead is creating a series of habits that will provide the foundation for healthy, satisfying eating.

The reason these core four principles work—my 2 Bunnies, as I call them, and you'll see why in my first video—is that it's just two simple things to remember when it comes to food and two small behavioral habits to do daily.

Eat and be accountable for what you eat. That's it. And it comes down to these four practices:

- **Water First:** Drink two glasses before every meal.
- **Veggies Most:** Fill half your plate with them.
- **The Scale:** Weigh yourself daily.
- **Track:** Hold yourself accountable.

When you do these four things, you will have allowed the 2B Mindset to lead you on a path to a lower weight and better body. Starting with this mindset will set you up to do other things well, too. You'll eat better, you'll know how to make good decisions, and you'll beat the temptation demons that like to rear their ugly heads every now and then.

I've always believed that successful weight loss is partly about what's on your plate, but it's mostly about what's in your mind. And that's what 2B Mindset is about—helping you shift from the traditional (and ultimately unsuccessful) ways you've looked at weight loss to a healthy and successful way to do it.

So let's take a look at how and why they work—and how you can get started the 2B way!

CORE 1

WATER FIRST

EVER SINCE I was young, I wanted a career in nutrition. Not only was it because of my personal struggle and relationships with food and the desire to help other people, but it was also because I was fascinated with the science of food. The macronutrients, the micronutrients, the way that they all interact and influence the body. After all, our foods do have the power to heal us, comfort us and fuel our bodies so we can optimize our health in so many ways.

But I also know that those of us who struggle or have struggled with weight aren't typically thinking about the science of nutrition or the ideal balance of foods—how many grams of this, how many ounces of that. We're concerned with the bottom line: How does it taste and make me feel—not just in the moment but also *after* I've eaten it? So the nutritional components are important, yes, but the relationship with all of our sources of food is even more so.

That's one of the reasons the first core principle in the 2B Mindset lays the foundation for shifting your entire way of thinking about food.

"Water First" is all about taking advantage of the simplest—yet perhaps most powerful—form of nutrition we have.

The simple fact is that most people don't drink enough water throughout the day, even though it is *the* secret weapon for dropping the pounds and feeling better overall, and really shouldn't be that much of a secret. To me, water is really the igniter switch to your whole weight-loss approach. Why?

- ■ *It makes you full*—so you're less likely to give in to cravings, to overeat at meals, and to allow temptation to override your mindset. This is key, as it works like a nutritional voice of reason, helping you make better decisions throughout the day. Here's one way to visualize it: Take a

16-ounce water bottle in your hand and place it on your other hand,
palm up, to see how naturally heavy it feels. Did it make your hand sink
a bit? That really demonstrates the point that water adds a nice
heaviness to the stomach, which gives you a sense of calm and satisfaction before eating your food, which also helps create a healthier
relationship with food.

■ *It helps you lose weight.* A study published in the *American Journal
of Clinical Nutrition* showed that drinking more water reduced
body weight after three months. And those who drank half a liter of
water (which is about half of a 2B Mindset bottle) lost 12 percent (or
4 pounds) more than the group that didn't. Another study shows that
drinking half a liter of water 30 minutes before each meal resulted in
a 44 percent greater weight loss.

■ *It helps quiet our hunger and settle those growls in our stomachs.*
Want to learn something cool? Our digestive tract is a super long and
windy system, about 30 feet long, in fact! It is not a straight slide from
your mouth to your bum, but instead, a roller coaster maze of curves
and turns. To help the food pass along the tract, it doesn't rely on
gravity but on contracting muscular movements that help vibrate the
food and waste along. This process is always working in a normal,
functioning body. What's interesting is when there are liquid and food
in the system, we can sometimes hear and feel these motions and
process them as hunger growls. Yet, if you feel that sense and then
drink a lot of water, it can help absorb the vibration and reduce that
sense of hunger. Try it! So if you claim you're "starving" and the first
thing you see are doughnuts, you don't want your eyes and mouth to
say, "Doughnuts!" You want them to say, "Water first!" Drink some
water, and you'll take the edge off—keeping you, or delaying you,
from eating something you don't necessarily need or want.

■ *It has many other health benefits,* potentially helping you fight
off headaches, according to research in the *European Journal
of Neurology,* and improve your mood, according to a study in the
journal *Appetite.*

- *It can also help stoke your metabolism,* if you drink cold water. Studies in the journal *Obesity* and the *International Journal of Obesity* show that drinking cold water can provide a small boost to assist with your natural fat-burning processes.

- *It's distracting.* While your new mindset is all about a new sense of focus, don't underestimate the power of distracting your mind, your mouth, even your hands—allowing you to form new habits (of drinking water), rather than relying on old ones (grabbing bags of chips, bowls of dips and anything else you like on your lips).

Ilana-ism

Two Hands on the Wheel

If you're in a situation with lots of snacks and appetizers around, I always say get your "two hands on the wheel" of your glass or water bottle!

The more water you drink, the more weight you may lose.
Here are the guidelines:

- *Drink half your weight in ounces, at a minimum, every day.* Turn this into your daily goal. A 150-pound person would drink 75 ounces (or about 9 glasses of water or 2½ 2B Mindset water bottles). A 200-pound person would have 100 ounces (or a little more than 12 glasses).

- *Aim to drink 16 ounces (480 ml) before every meal.* That even means before you have a cup of coffee. Water First, Water First, Water First. This will give your stomach a chance to say, "Hang on, we don't need to eat that whole cheese tray right now." Try to drink between 5 and 20 minutes before every meal.

  Keep your 2B Mindset water bottle handy to remind yourself to hit your daily water goal. Very soon, this new habit will become automatic—and you'll see it in the benefits.

CORE 2

VEGGIES MOST

O NE OF THE greatest things that you get with the 2B Mindset is this: Power.

Power over your choices. Power over your body. Power to make changes that can give you energy, help you lose weight and make you feel better every single day. This power comes in many forms—emotional, psychological and nutritional.

So when we talk about nutritional power, we have to start with nature's most potent player when it comes to weight loss and your overall health.

"Veggies Most" works because of all of the benefits that come from vegetables. Packed with fiber, they help make you feel full, and that's partly what helps with greater results in weight loss. A 12-month randomized controlled trial published in the *European Journal of Clinical Nutrition* showed that eating more vegetables led to greater hunger satisfaction, meaning it made people feel less hungry (weight loss was related to the amount of calories coming from vegetables). So the more vegetables people were consuming, the greater weight loss results they were seeing. Another study published in the *American Journal of Clinical Nutrition* showed that advising people to eat big volumes of low-calorie foods like veggies and soups was a more successful weight-loss strategy than advising people to restrict their portions and focus on eating less.

Vegetables also contain vitamins, minerals and other compounds that are repeatedly shown to keep you at your healthiest. And when I refer to "veggies," I am talking about the lower-calorie veggies—like eggplant, spaghetti squash, bell peppers and cucumber—that you'll be wanting to eat in volume, as opposed to starchier vegetables like potatoes and corn. (I'll go through the complete run-down of their nutritional benefits in the next chapter.) These are the best way to fill your stomach without making it grow.

Veggie Myths Busted

- *"Aren't vegetables going to be expensive and high-maintenance?"* You can help reduce costs by buying frozen veggies (or in bulk) or finding veggies on sale. For example, cabbage is a very budget friendly vegetable because you can usually find it year round, it lasts a while in your fridge and is very inexpensive and supremely versatile. And if you're looking for ease of preparation, try frozen vegetables, or ones that are pre-cut.

- *"What about potatoes and corn—are they veggies or carbs?"* I consider those foods fiber-filled carbs (FFCs) because they have more than 50 calories per cup. By the 2B definition, veggies are much lower in starch and carbohydrates and higher in water while also being packed with fiber. Some varieties of squash, like butternut squash, are also on the FFC list. The only exception to the 50-calorie line is beets. (The American Diabetes Association considers beets a non-starchy vegetable, and I've never seen anyone overeat or gain weight from them, have you?)

- *"What about tomatoes and carrots?"* You may have been told that carrots are higher in sugar, but carrots have about 50 calories per cup, and I've never seen a client or myself gain weight from them. I highly encourage you to try, track and see for yourself that avoiding carrots likely leads to more weight gain than eating lots and lots of them. While tomatoes are technically a fruit, they're certainly considered a veggie the way they are prepared (and they also have fewer than 50 calories per cup).

The "Veggies Most" way of thinking applies to your overall approach to eating: Every meal, just make sure that most of your plate is filled with vegetables (they're extra credit at breakfast!).

Plant-based power is your nutritional backbone. But we also need to be real here. Vegetables do have an image problem. We know they're good for you, but we often take them for granted. And the truth is, we just don't see them with the same culinary sexiness as crème brulée or pasta parmigiana.

We all need to change the narrative. In some circles, vegetables have a bad rap: boring, tasteless, yuck.

Wrong, wrong, wrong.

If you speak to any fit, happy and healthy person over 35 years old maintaining an ideal size, you'll likely hear their enthusiasm for different dishes, recipes and tips straight away.

Veggies can be as delicious and savory as your favorite meal to indulge in (you'll see how in the recipes!). So to get to the place where "Veggies Most" becomes second nature, you need to shift to the 2B Mindset. And you will see: The more meals that include "Veggies Most," the more weight you will lose.

These are some ways to think about veggies that can help you elevate veggies from a supporting role to a leading one.

Veggies Are the New Comfort Food: The words "comfort food" (in conversation or in hashtags) usually conjure up the same images— Nana's lasagna, a pint of ice cream, deep dish pizza, or some other heavy dish. They're called that because, in the moment, they make you feel better as they load your belly and satisfy cravings for salt, fat, sugar or size. The only problem with too many of those comfort foods is that they're often the source of discomfort—sometimes because of how you feel after eating them and sometimes because they can be part of what contributes to your weight gain and poor health. While you'll still be able to enjoy those foods from time to time with the 2B Mindset, I think it's time we redefined what "comfort" means.

- *Comfort foods should make you feel satisfied.*

- *Comfort foods should not make you feel guilty.*

- *Comfort foods should do your body more good than harm.*

- *Comfort foods should make you feel like you can go out and see people after.*

- *Comfort foods should make you happy (and comfortable in your pants!).*

- *Veggies—when you know how to make them in quick, savory, yummy and exciting ways—hit all of those checkmarks.*

Ilana-ism

A Healthy Outside Starts from the Inside.

When you eat better you start to feel better.

Focus, Focus, Focus: I know that this may not be easy at first. If you're low on veggie consumption, it can be difficult to just flip a switch and change the ratio of your typical meal plate. Maybe it's out of habit, and maybe it's because you don't always have easy access to vegetables. The only way to approach that is through focus. Yes, it takes planning. It takes a commitment to the "Veggies Most" principle. It takes thinking about your vegetable consumption until it becomes second nature.

Remember, this isn't a diet plan, so there's no counting, no weighing, no specific meals you have to have. And that's what makes this relatively simple and straightforward: Drink your water and fill your plate with vegetables. Win that game, and you'll win the ultimate one.

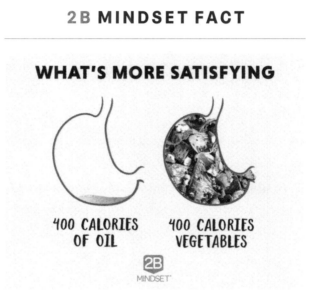

2B MINDSET FACT

WHAT'S MORE SATISFYING

400 CALORIES OF OIL   **400 CALORIES VEGETABLES**

2B MINDSET

When you look at 400 calories of a high-fat food (something oily like fries or chips) compared to 400 calories of veggies, you can see how much room the veggies take up in your stomach. The high-fat foods take up much less space, leaving you hungry and unsatisfied, which tends to result in you eating more and more.

Find Your Favorites: Green, white, red, yellow, orange. Leafy, crunchy, squishy. Veggies come in all shapes, sizes, flavors and textures—and there's one (or many) for you. As you're working on "Veggies Most," find the few that you really like and make them a staple. It can be broccoli, cauliflower, squash or peppers. Whatever your veggie lovin' (or soon-to-be veggie lovin') heart desires. We will talk about this more in the next chapter, because for ongoing weight loss, it's important not only to have veggies that you can stomach, but also to have a few that you genuinely crave and enjoy. That way, you always know you have something on hand to fill your plate. And remember, these can come in all forms—raw, frozen, canned, grilled, flavored with any hundreds of spices or accessories (see Chapter 6). Just as long as you have your go-to veggies, you'll never have to guess, scramble or go without.

Experimentation with Vegetation: As I promised, I'm not going to talk about math much at all when it comes to the 2B Mindset. No counting calories or grams or measuring portions. But if you'll forgive me for just a few sentences, I want you to consider this math: You have dozens of vegetables, dozens of spices, dozens of herbs and dozens of cooking methods. The statistical conclusion: There are thousands of different ways to prepare vegetables. The combinations are endless, and that means the possibilities are, too. So while your lifestyle has to dictate what you're able to do, I do want to encourage you to act like your own mad scientist—try different combinations to come up with whatever your tongue desires (savory, spicy, salty, even sweet?). But if you don't feel creative, that's okay. I've come up with many, many recipes and simple dishes to give you ideas for amazing tasting veggies. This ability to make up so many different combinations of flavors will go a long way in helping you redefine veggies as the new comfort food.

Control Your Place, Control Your Plate: Here's the thing about just about every diet plan out there. It all sounds well and good *until*.... *Until* your significant other suggests a special night out at a new place that everybody is raving about... *Until* your friends say it's been a long time since everyone got together and "Hey, how about drinks tonight?"... *Until* the office party... *Until* you're on the road... Until, until, until.... "Until" has derailed more diets than chips and soda.

So how do you handle it? Certainly, the 2B water-veggie combination will help you through many of those situations, but oftentimes, it's all about trying to find ways to control the situation. What do I mean? If your group suggests going to the Korean barbecue place, maybe you can suggest going for sushi or Chinese instead (more options for veggies). There's nothing wrong with living and socializing and having foods you love, but make a point to dictate what you want the environment to be (ordering fajitas with lots of veggies at the Mexican place, rather than the triple-burrito special). Tell yourself that no matter what the environment, you *can* control it.

Ultimately, a "Veggies Most" mindset is the key nutritional principle that will steer your weight loss in the right direction. Plant power is real power. Plant power is *your* power.

Ilana-ism

Every Color Has Plant Power

All veggies are packed with nutrients, enzymes and phytonutrients that benefit all of our bodily processes. Greens are great but they are not alone. Orange veggies like carrots are great sources for Vitamin A; red bell peppers have Vitamin C, if you're looking for some immune support; spinach is a source of iron and broccoli is a good source of calcium.

CORE 3

THE SCALE

'VE WORKED WITH enough people to know that many people who struggle with weight have a very complicated relationship with the scale. It's a source of frustration (when you feel like you do everything right, but don't achieve the goals you want). It's a source of anger (how did *this* happen?). It's a blind spot (maybe if I just don't step on it, I won't have to feel guilty about the double order of fries?). Plus, the scale is commonly perceived as the mouthy teenager—it just loves to taunt, tease and talk back to you.

We love to hate it, mostly because of all of those emotions wrapped up in wherever the number falls.

We need to, however, learn to love it.

And I don't say that in an "embrace who you are" kind of way. I say that in a very straightforward way. Your weight is a data point. Your weight is *the* key data point. How do you know where you are, how far you have to go and how far you've been without knowing your data?

I tell people all the time to think of teachers. A teacher works with a classroom full of students. They don't all just sit there and think about the world. The teacher gives assessments—tests, quizzes, essays, you name it—to evaluate how much a student has learned and processed.

The scale is your test—your accountability measure (students would never do the work if they didn't have that accountability; the same could be said for people trying to lose weight—easy to give up when there's no accountability). The scale communicates to you important lessons about your habits, about what can work for you and about what can help.

That tends to be one of the biggest changes for many people

adopting the 2B Mindset. They go from rarely using the scale to learning from it every day. But it works. Why? Many reasons, no doubt. Here's one of the biggest: Instead of thinking that the scale is shaming you, you should think of it like a quiet coach—informing you, teaching you, nudging you, motivating you and guiding you. When you flip this data point from something that's often thought of as a negative and start thinking of it as a positive, you open a whole new world of learning about yourself—and better equip yourself to make decisions that will have a positive influence on your weight.

I know that it might not be so easy. For so long, the scale was like the "unknown caller" that pops up on our phone; it's pretty easy to ignore. But I know I can make it easier for you, as I have with the thousands of people who have the 2B Mindset. On top of accountability, it also instills a sense of urgency. Think about paying taxes, something no one really wants to do. If you didn't have them pulled out of your monthly paycheck, or the threat of an IRS audit, or an April fifteenth deadline, how easy would it be to push off payment or skip it altogether?

Here's the bottom line, really: Your weight is the essence of what you want to change. You may be motivated by fitness goals, overall health improvement, or having more energy, but if you're covered in excess pounds, how truly possible are those results? And in order to address weight gain, you have to deal directly with the data. It's crazy not to. Think about what happens with a two-pound weight gain, which could easily happen with a night of nachos. *Two pounds is no big deal, right?* You probably won't even notice it—and you won't if you're not weighing yourself daily. But what happens if you avoid the scale and that two pounds becomes 30, or 50, or more? Instead of just monitoring your weight on a $20 tool that you keep in your bathroom, you now have to wear new clothes, take medications and increase your risk of heart attack, all because you avoided the scale.

2B MINDSET SUCCESS STORY

*Micki F., an Independent Team Beachbody Coach, 50, New York, New York, lost 26 pounds in 5 months**

"Journaling every day showed me exactly where my problem was."

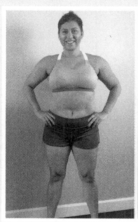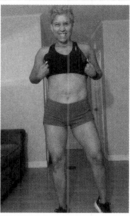

Results vary depending on starting point and effort.

T IS SCIENTIFICALLY proven that metabolism slows down as we age, making it harder to keep weight off. However, you never have to accept weight gain as a normal part of the aging process. Take Micki for example. In the years leading up to her fiftieth birthday, she gained 30 pounds and didn't feel comfortable in her own skin. Additionally, her cholesterol level kept getting higher. "I was scared to end up with high blood pressure like my parents, who both suffered strokes," she admits.

Journaling is an incredibly important part of the 2B Mindset program, and was crucial to Micki's transformation. "Journaling every day showed me exactly where my problem was. I had been eating my issues instead of facing them," she says. "I no longer stress out if I see a pound or two increase on the scale because I know exactly what needs to be done to reverse it."

Here's how to approach the scale—and make it work for you.

Weigh yourself daily first thing in the morning: Ideally, you want to get on the scale after you wake up, right after you go to the bathroom. And you should not have eaten for about ten hours beforehand. This "dry" weight will give you the most consistency from day to day and help you better track your progress. (Note: If you're a shift worker, follow the same pattern; weigh yourself after you wake up and haven't had food, even if that's two p.m.—not in the morning.)

One of the biggest questions I get is this: Why do you have to do it daily instead of weekly?

I've worked with thousands and thousands of people. Even before working with Beachbody, I've seen hundreds of private clients and led a weight-loss seminar at UCLA for hundreds of employees. I used to not recommend daily weigh-ins. I used to recommend just a minimum of Mondays and Fridays, because Monday tells us what happened over the weekend, and Friday tells us what happened over the week. But what I found in speaking with people who wanted to stick to once a week—because they were used to that from Weight Watchers or someone else telling them that—their mindset was fixated on the weigh-in day.

Anyone who tells me they did Weight Watchers, I ask, "What's your day?" Meaning, what's their weigh-in day. It's usually the first thing they remember about the experience, far more so than if I ask them to recall what they were eating day to day while on the program. So if your day is Friday, then you feel like Friday night you can go crazy, have your cocktails, have your chocolate, no worries. You're not getting on the scale for a week. And then Saturday is still kind of sloppy. Sunday, too. You get it into gear Monday and crash-diet for another Friday, and the cycle continues.

Why is this bad? I see people manipulate their food that way and cause unhealthy relationships with it because they're eating and not fully enjoying it. It reinforces the dieting mentality and treats eating for your body like this on-and-off game. Friday night was permission night, rather than just fully enjoying what you want when you want it and being present with that food. I found that people who are going on a scale once a week were actually manipulating their food and playing more of a game with it than anything.

Another reason I dislike the weekly approach is that if you're working hard and sticking to Veggies Most a lot of the week, making healthy choices and swapping the cocktail for sparkling water (while your friends are getting drunk), then you do a weigh-in and it stays the same, you'll feel defeated. You'll feel like, "I've been doing such a good job! WTF!"

When you weigh yourself daily, you'll establish patterns of what is working and what isn't so you can better figure out what you want to do more consistently and what you actually don't want to do as often.

This consistency will condition you to have a better relationship with the scale, so you don't freak out if things aren't totally going your way.

You don't need anything fancy: I have a $25 scale that I bought from Amazon. I know a lot of people who have fancy scales that measure body-fat percentage, but those are highly inaccurate and not necessary. You just need one point of data: your weight.

Simply, it works: Much research points to the fact that weighing yourself regularly is one of the key components for having weight-loss success. In the National Weight Control Registry (a group of more than 10,000 people who have lost an average of 66 pounds and kept it off for five or more years), the habits of these people are tracked. So this is all about the people who have lost weight and kept it off. Nearly

80 percent of those people weigh themselves regularly. A large review of studies published in SAGE Open found a correlation between frequency of weighing and weight loss and maintenance. And one study in the *American Journal of Health Behavior* showed that 46 percent of people were successful at weight loss when they weighed in weekly, compared to only 8 percent who didn't use the scale. And when you consider the fight that we all have—living in a society that promotes obesity through TV, radio, billboards, social media and more—this is quite an accomplishment. Not to mention it's the simplest tool you can use to fight against the multi-billion-dollar industries that have a vested interest in wanting you *not* to lose weight.

Ilana-ism
Think Two Pounds at a Time

I said it in Chapter 1 and I'm saying it again here. For many people, expectations about weight loss are way too high. If you're focused on losing ten pounds by a reunion or a wedding and the scale isn't moving, you freak out. Or you know that you have 100 pounds to lose, or 50 pounds, or 20 pounds, and the scale is not moving, so you go nuts. Bring it back down to two pounds at a time, and it will start to move. If you're focused on too big of a number, it's going to completely overwhelm you. Focus on two pounds—or even two ounces—and it will give you more momentum to realize the scale is actually moving.

It may surprise you: Here's a common misconception that people have about weight loss—that it can't happen on the weekends (not with the parties and pizza, the brunch and booze). But with the 2B Mindset, you might see that the weekends actually bring you better weight loss, and that's why I love going on the scale daily and not just once a week. If you're only going on the scale once a week, you might think something like, *I don't know what is holding me back from losing the weight.* But when you're on the scale daily, you actually may see movement on the weekend, even though you weren't expecting it. Maybe it was because you slept in more, are less stressed, aren't sitting around as much, or don't eat out of anxiety (because you're less stressed). A lot of people lose more weight on the weekends, and the scale can help you figure out what's working.

Also, we live in a world now where you couldn't avoid dieting advice and food marketing if you tried. While someone may have told you that red meat is bad for you, you may see perfectly clearly that sliced lean steak flocked with a plate of Veggies Most gets you losing weight and in better overall shape. You will be shocked at how much simpler the overall process can be.

Avoiding it is working against you: If you think about a time you've gained weight—whether it was after you had a kid or got to a desk job or coming off an injury—you probably know what the trigger was that led you onto that path. But you probably haven't broken down all the variables that went into that weight gain. One of those variables, I would bet, is that every time you gained a decent amount of weight, you avoided the scale. That avoidance—the equivalent of covering your eyes and singing, "I can't see it, I can't see it"—contributed to it, because you could "ignore" the wake-up call the scale would have been trying to give you. This all becomes part of the negative relationship we have with the scale—you feel like you have to do crazy things to see the number go down, which isn't the case.

You'll learn to go with the flow, not be derailed by fluctuations: A lot of you will see amazing success and drop a ton of weight early. You'll drop a pound or two and then you'll see the scale go up by a few ounces. When you have a negative relationship with the scale, your immediate reaction may be to throw in the towel (or throw it out the window) and get negative. But when you weigh yourself daily, you'll quickly shift your mindset. The scale won't be taunting or scolding or mocking you for enjoying that glass of wine. It will simply be giving you information. It's just feedback. You're always either losing weight or learning, and that's a very powerful concept to embrace.

When I'm Losing Weight, I Love...

MYSELF FOR STAYING STRONG.

MY BODY FOR SHOWING THE RESULTS.

MY FAMILY AND FRIENDS FOR RECOGNIZING ME.

MY SCALE FOR ACCOUNTABILITY.

You can celebrate non-scale victories, too: Not everyone loves the scale. Personal trainers tend to be the most prominent people who tell you to throw out the scale, saying that weight isn't the only measure of fitness. I remember going to personal trainers when I was 100 pounds heavier, and they would say, "Don't look at the scale, go by how you feel." For me, someone who was sitting in a body with 100 pounds of excess weight, I didn't feel different day-to-day, and I wasn't in tune with my body at all. I could eat three bags of chips or three bags of salad—my problem was I kept eating. So I needed that scale for feedback and for information. Feel can only get you so far—because you may not feel every effect, positive or negative, at least not immediately. You need an objective tool to help you really track what's working and what's not.

You may feel that your car is driving smoothly, but when you glance at the dashboard, it's telling you that you need more gas and an oil change.

But this doesn't mean you should ignore non-scale victories. Is it easier to walk up stairs? Are you able to lift heavier weights? Are your clothes fitting better? Are your inches getting smaller? Every victory matters.

During my 100-pound weight loss, it was a very big deal when I was able to shop in clothing stores that weren't classified as "plus size." That was a big "plus," so to speak—but it took about 25 or 35 pounds to get there. Not having "chub rub" in my thighs—another huge non-scale victory, because chub rub is brutal—took another 25 pounds. Being able to cross my legs: huge non-scale victory. Being able to wear a dress: victory. Being able to work out without huffing and puffing. There are so many. But unfortunately, it takes some time to get to these celebratory wins. You will like when you can celebrate two pounds at a time. You'll have ongoing successes and feel proud, excited and motivated along the process.

The scale is THE tool that will help you customize your nutrition: When people start going on the scale daily, they start to create their own system, they start to trust themselves, treat themselves and not feel like they're cheating themselves. They start to realize that they actually can lose weight eating normally and being human. You'll do this in so many ways, such as:

- ***Referring to your tracker:*** If the scale is down a pound in the morning, you can refer to yesterday's tracker page as a weight-loss day. That's great, and you want to pin that and get excited about that. But if it goes up, learn from it. Don't be reactive, don't be hostile. You can absolutely always lose weight just as fast as you can gain weight. So if you can gain half a pound in a day, you can also lose half a pound in a day. If you could gain a full pound in a day, you can lose a full pound in a day. You always have to tell yourself that, "I could always lose it as fast as I could gain it." Take a deep breath, and refer to your tracker to give you the clues as to what works for you.

- *Noting trends:* You'll learn from how much water you drink, how many veggies you have and other patterns as they relate to what you see on the scale. If you have 10, 20, 30 pounds or more to lose, it's going to take some time—and the scale won't go down every day. Sometimes you need the scale to go up to learn what causes it to go up, and that will help reshape your mindset about what you want to crave and have more often, and what isn't really worth it, and question why did you even have that silly thing in the first place?

- *Figuring out your system:* Weight loss actually gets better, easier and more effective as you figure out your system. How much protein should you have? Can you have six meatballs or should you just stick to four? How do I know if a potato will help or hurt me? We're all so different, which is why you have to see what the scale is telling you, so you can adjust your eating to what has positive results for you.

Before You Start, Get a Physical. *I personally recommend, as a dietitian, that everyone gets a physical before starting the 2B Mindset. Get your blood checked. Have a good starting point with that. Because that's also a really beautiful part of this program: your overall health and well-being can improve. You can track that kind of data in your journal, should you wish.*

You will learn to love it: Honestly, some people freak out that I promote the scale so much. In the first three days of the program, you may be like, "Ilana is a witch making me go on the scale!"

After a few weeks you'll likely become obsessed with it. Have a cookie or cocktail and see the number go up by only 0.1 or 0.2 or not even at all, and you learn that it's not so scary—that you don't have to derail your way of eating just because you deviate a little from time to time. In the same way you see what makes it go up, you learn what makes it go down. Perhaps the greatest strength of using the scale is that it can be a really nice wake-up call to emotional eating—and showing that it's more destructive than productive.

If you hate it now, that's okay—that's normal. But when you trust the process, you'll decrease the anxiety around food and your weight.

Use it daily, but think about it long-term: Because your weight will always fluctuate day to day—thanks to your hormones, or too much salt or a too-late dinner. It could also be because of constipation or swollen muscles from intense exercise. So it really takes zooming out and getting a better perspective. It takes looking at the scale more sensibly and logically. Day-to-day accountability has the huge dividends I've described here, but the real victory comes from looking at what is happening week-to-week and in your overall progress.

The payoff: You will have a better relationship with food. Part of the reason is that you can actually have a slice of cake or a glass of wine, and as long as all the other principles are in check, you'll be okay. Sometimes you'll even see a weight loss the next day. Or it might stay the same. Or, your weight goes up 0.2 and you thought it was going to go up 15. That, really, is the key to having a better relationship with food.

A lot of people feel that if they have a piece of cake, they might as well eat the whole cake—and the bag of chips. That is the culture we live in—might as well eat the whole pizza if I have one slice. The scale teaches you that you can have something without destroying everything. And you start to realize that food isn't as scary as we've made it.

Instead of demonizing the scale, embracing it will give you more freedom and flexibility—so you can stop thinking that food is so dangerous. Thinking of food as poison and/or cutting out everything— that's not very sustainable. But when you see that you could actually have these things, but in a smarter approach, you'll notice the scale won't change much. Your body's still beautiful. You just need the right mindset.

The Number Isn't Enough. *Yes, you'll be using the scale daily. But I want you also to add a physical goal to provide a real-life check on your weight gain and weight loss. Maybe it's getting into your wedding dress. Maybe it's feeling comfortable in a bathing suit. Maybe it's looking good in photos at your cousin's bar mitzvah, or running a half marathon, or wanting your doctor to reveal your blood pressure and cholesterol levels have lowered. Pick one you care about the most. The number on the scale alone is not enough.*

CORE 4

TRACK

So now that you're committed to weighing yourself daily (and understanding all of the benefits of doing so), the question remains: What are you going to do with that data?

You could react to it emotionally, for better or worse. You could stow it away in a deep corner of your brain. Or you could just step on the scale, close your eyes and pretend you did the deed.

But you're not. You're going to use that data for what it is: Data. Information. Feedback.

The fourth component of the 2B Mindset is that your weight-loss journey isn't just about going through the motions of what someone tells you to do. It's taking the feedback you're getting, learning from it and making necessary adjustments. The only way you can do that is through tracking key points of data, such as what you eat, when you eat, your weight and how you feel. When you do so, you will see trends, and you will notice what has profound effects on your weight, energy, mood and more.

This is why tracking is so crucial. The only way to make adjustments is to make them based on *your* data—what your body is telling you based on the foods you eat and your common behaviors. The best part is that this won't involve hours and hours of data collection. No spreadsheets, no pesky calculations, no crazy time commitment.

The three keys for tracking:

- Every day, complete a "My Day" page in your book or track on the Beachbody app. Go to the app store on your mobile device and search for "Beachbody."

- You bite it, write it. Drink it, ink it. After your meal and water, track it. Build this habit and you will be golden. To help you master it, take out your cell phone. Every phone now is armed with an alarm clock. Set up three: one for ten a.m. titled, "Today's a great day, drink water and track"; one for two p.m. that says, "Doing great, fill up and track"; and one for nine p.m. that says, "Get ready for bed and track your day."

■ You can choose how detailed you want to be. The more information you input, the more insight you have into what works for you—and what will empower you to stay on track. It should take no more than five minutes a day to log what you eat and when. But I would recommend that you be as detailed as possible. Just writing "nut butter" or "bread" in your tracker usually won't cut it. There's a very big difference between a teaspoon, a tablespoon and a giant, globbing spoon of peanut butter when you're trying to lose weight. And just writing "bread" won't give you the future insight that "one thick slice of sourdough" will.

■ Be honest. If you eat it or drink it, track it. The feedback is designed to help you, so there's no advantage to lying or hiding information. You will see direct correlations between what you eat and weight changes from day to day. It will become some of the most important data you use as you learn to customize and adjust your habits and what you eat. And record how you're feeling, too. Writing when you're stressed, for example, will give you greater insight into your eating behaviors.

As you track, you should keep these three truths in mind.

We're all different: Some kids learn how to walk at eight months, and some kids learn how to walk at 18 months. But at the end of the day, do we all know how to walk? It's a life skill. Same thing with eating well and learning how to control your weight in the way that best suits your life. So be patient and figure out how to walk, so to speak. You will feel absolutely amazing and empowered when you learn how to eat to control your weight. While some people appear to manage their weight easily, it's just a fact that they figured it out earlier and have stayed consistent with it, but that's why tracking is so crucial. It provides the building blocks of feedback that help you learn and maintain this life skill. But what works for your friend may not be the right fit for you. So more than anything, keep in mind that *your* data will show *you* where you can make changes or tweaks that can have big effects on *your own* weight loss.

Spend some time with the feedback: Instead of asking such things as whether you should have one slice of bread or two, why not try it and see what effect each has? Some people may be fine with two; others work better with one. I'm not suggesting that you just always default to one slice because it's fewer than two. Instead, just try it out for yourself, track it, and see what happens. Then learn from it, so you know what's best for you next time. Some people may gain weight when they have two slices of bread, and others may lose weight when they have two because it gives them better energy and they eat better throughout the day. You need to go in with an open mind, because this is about to be the most freeing and successful approach to weight loss you will ever experience. Try it, track it, and see for yourself.

Learn from the clock, not just the plate: At the last minute, I decided that we needed to include a "time" entry in the tracker book. That's because time can play a big role in weight loss. Some people find earlier dinners help with weight loss, while others learn that having a snack at a certain time of day really helps. Logging your time in the tracker is what's going to get you realizing what works best for you. This can also be helpful for logging your exercise, since you may notice patterns about energy and weight loss depending on when you do or don't eat before or after your workouts.

The 2B Mindset starts with these four core principles—Water First, Veggies Most, the Scale and Tracking. They will get you started on a journey that ultimately helps improve your relationship with food, your mind, and your body; and help you customize your habits and eating patterns to eat the best way that works for you, your tastes and your lifestyle.

And when you do these four things, you will see the success—in plain sight. Drink that water and eat those veggies, then let your scale and your tracker tell you all you need to know and exactly what you need to hear.

Ilana-ism

If You Can Scroll, You Can Track

Please don't say you don't have time to track. It takes three to five minutes a day. (Some research shows that the average person spends about two hours on social media a day! If you've got time for that, you've got time to track.)

CHAPTER SUMMARY

■ *The Core Four foundational principles of 2B Mindset are: Water First (drink two glasses before every meal), Veggies Most (fill half your plate with them), the Scale (weigh yourself daily) and Track (hold yourself accountable).*

■ *Water makes you full, helps you lose weight, quiets your hunger, stokes your metabolism and has many other health benefits. Drink two glasses before every meal.*

■ *Veggies make you feel full, are packed with fiber and essential nutrients, can be a comfort food and you can eat a ton while still losing weight. Fill up half your plate with them at lunch and dinner.*

■ *The scale tells you where you are and how far you have to go. Weigh yourself first thing in the morning. The more often you get on the scale, usually the less of a "thing" it becomes.*

■ *Track your progress—noting what you eat, when you eat it and how you feel—every day. You bite it, you write it. When you do this, you'll notice how food affects your weight, energy and mood.*

A NEW WAY TO LOOK AT FOOD GROUPS

Discover How Eating for Weight Loss
Leads to Better Choices—and Success.

WHEN YOU'VE SPENT the number of hours I've
spent with clients and people who have struggled with their weight, you have heard everything.
After all, the diet industry is full of so many variations, plans and programs that claim to help you lose weight if you can
just follow the rules.

Right? You hear me, because you've probably tried or know of so
many of these variations. Bust the sugar, ditch the carbs, feast on fat.
Eat these recipes for 30 days. Fast for 18 hours. Eat clean. Eat and
cheat. Measure this. Count that. Lock your fridge to protect against

the midnight crazies. The problem is that extreme diets get marketed as sexy and are great for businesses to make a lot of money, but what's actually great for your health, we all know, is moderation, which is hard to achieve without practicing the Core Four and acquiring the 2B Mindset. With all of the noise that's around us—between the ads that coax us to dive into buckets of fried chicken to information that seems to contradict itself from one day to the next—it's no wonder so many people struggle, gain weight and then feel stuck in a place that they can't seem to get out of.

But when you adopt the 2B Mindset, you'll see that food doesn't control you, eating doesn't have to be an all-or-nothing proposition, and what and how you eat isn't meant to be an impulsive response to emotions and advertisements.

Eating is about knowledge. Eating is about striking the perfect balance between pleasure and fuel. Eating is about control and requires customization. Eating is about an approach—maybe even a swagger—to food that turns you from a victim of emotional eating and your food environment to a proactive commander (and lover) of your personal eating style. When it comes to books, movies, art and music, you are someone who knows what you like. You know what works and are in tune with what satisfaction for you is all about. And you must know, there is no one perfect way to eat. So you design the perfect way for you.

The 2B Mindset doesn't tell you what you should eat through a detailed prescription of ingredients or recipes (though I have plenty that I am sharing with you, and I am constantly adding to The Mindset Membership to give you endless ideas for delicious meals you will love). Instead, it helps you learn about what you should eat and why. Once you have that knowledge, you'll be in full control of what you eat every day.

Why is this so crucial? When it comes to weight loss, food is *everything*. I know we live in a grit-and-grind exercise culture—and there are many benefits to exercise—but the big battle over weight is *always* won or lost with nutrition.

But for me to imply that any one formula will work for every single person would simply be misleading at best and dead wrong at worst.

You have to find what works for *you*.

When you embrace that concept, you will unlock so many of the handcuffs that have been holding you back on your weight-loss journey.

This journey should start with learning how food works—and how to make it work in your favor.

In this chapter, I will take you through a new way of thinking about food groups and how to approach eating. With that knowledge (and by following the Core Four principles of the 2B Mindset from the previous chapter), you'll be equipped with everything you need to start watching the number on the scale go down consistently.

First, I do think it's important to briefly look at the big picture—the role of food, how it interacts with your body and the science of weight gain and loss. These are the key concepts and terms I think it's just kinda cool to know about:

Macronutrients

These are the main sources of energy found in foods—protein, carbohydrates and fat. Specific foods are typically not one macronutrient, but a combination of them—for example, nuts, which contain all three, and meat, which can be high in both protein and fat. Given the confusing and calculating nature of "macros," I've created four main categories of food that you will see below.

Micronutrients

These are the elements that we need in smaller quantities, like vitamins and minerals, which tend to be notably abundant in fruits and vegetables. They're essential for the operation of certain systems in your body, such as your immune system; however they're not something that necessarily motivates us and directs our food choices day to day.

Calories

You're all too familiar with these, but in simplest terms, a calorie is a unit of energy. We all burn calories daily just merely to live and breathe, and therefore require outside energy in the form of food calories to sustain our daily activities. When your calorie intake far exceeds your calorie output, you will likely gain weight. However, not all calories are created equal, and the quality of your food matters, despite the calorie value.

One gram of carbohydrates or protein contains 4 calories, while 1 gram of fat contains 9 calories. Because fat is denser in calories, consuming high fat and deep-fried foods is especially tricky for volume eaters who are looking to fill their stomachs.

When it comes to arming yourself with information about nutrition, it's also important to learn a bit about how your body uses, stores and burns food. I took advanced level classes in biology, microbiology, biochemistry and organic chemistry to better understand these nuanced and complex ideas and broke it down to the simplest form for you. When you understand the "why" behind "what" foods you should eat, it will help you so much.

Food, of course, serves as the body's nourishment. Everything in your body—from your muscles to your brain, from your kidneys to your eyeballs—needs energy in order to operate. Food serves as the power source for it all.

As soon as you put something in your mouth, that triggers the digestive process—the process that breaks down food into its nutrients and into the energy (remember calories are units of energy) that gets shuttled throughout your body for necessary use. In a perfect world, you'd have exactly the number of calories you'd need to operate, with perhaps just a little left over that could be stored as fat (that fat came in handy in our ancestors' days, so it could be cultivated as a source of backup energy).

Our modern way of living doesn't nearly simulate that state of equilibrium—as we often consume way more calories than we need to break down and use for energy. That's when your body can't keep up with the flood of calories and the increases in blood sugar. So the body packs them away as too much fat—your body's version of a storage closet. Imagine the gems you can find if you clear out the junk!

Careful with Calorie Counting

- Calorie counts can be off by 20 percent on packaged goods and restaurant food and still be legal. That 800-calorie cheeseburger could easily have closer to 950 calories.

- People underreport how many calories they consume by an average of 32 percent.

- Calories aren't equal. The nutrition of the food can impact whether or not it causes weight gain.

- Calorie counting may improve food awareness but can cause food anxiety. Counting down from a budgeted quantity throughout the day can put you in a scarcity mindset that leads to skipping meals in order to "save up" for binges later.

Now, so many variables can influence this process—whether it's your genetic disposition that governs your metabolism (the rate at which you use energy), the amount you burn through physical activity, or the kinds of foods you eat. That last factor is a variable because the body doesn't process every food the same way. For example, vegetables and other fiber-filled carbohydrates help stabilize blood sugar and stay in your digestive system longer, making you feel full and less likely to overeat. And simple carbohydrates, also known as sugar, which you'll find in too many foods these days, quickly flood your bloodstream with excess glucose—and have the propensity to be turned into fat because your body can't use them all at once.

So one of the main reasons why the 2B Mindset works is that, by taking control of your food and understanding how it interacts with your body, you'll learn how to tweak your choices to achieve a state where, essentially, you're burning more energy than you need, so that your body relies on your body fat to get energy. That decrease in your body fat helps you lose weight and gets you closer to a state where your body is working in sync—eating the right kinds and amounts of food, maintaining a healthy weight, and having the personal energy to feel great.

So now the question becomes: How do you get there?

In studying nutrition and food science for many years, I've found that it really breaks down to four basic food groups that you need to think about. I have also found through my work that instructions can't be overly complicated or limiting. They have to allow you to explore— and they have to make you feel good both when you're eating and when you've finished.

These four food groups will be what allows you to take control of your nutrition and think smarter about it. When you do that, that's when you start making food work for you and not against you.

VEGGIES: **MAKE THEM YOUR FOCUS**
Why: *They Make You Full and Satisfied*

AFTER YOU DRINK your Water First, eat Veggies Most. Always make a veggie your first bite. I'm not saying that because I want you to get them out of the way; I'm saying that because when you make veggies your first bite, you will always be more likely to eat more of them, which will help you lose more weight. When was the last time you started with pizza and fries and then went searching for a salad or minestrone soup? When you start with the veggie, you are always better off. And you will see later on how pizza and fries get incorporated, but a quick hint: It's after you've had your Veggies Most. Because this controls urges and temptations to overeat as well.

You can try high-fat diets like keto or high-protein diets like Atkins all you want, but from my research and experience, the only way to successfully stay slim long term is to learn to love veggies. When you study people who don't struggle with dieting and their weight, you will likely find they've eaten three to five different veggies in the last 24 hours. Not because they had to; because they've learned to want to. I find that your health can be determined by noting the five foods that you eat most; when veggies make their way on that list, you'll be amazed at how your weight and energy will improve.

Nutritionally, you can't get much better than veggies. As a reminder, I define veggies as low-starch veggies with 50 calories or fewer per cup. Think tomatoes, zucchini, eggplant, mushrooms, cucumbers, peppers, cabbage, carrots, spinach and broccoli. It's why I put so much stock in plant power. The main reasons why veggies serve as the key to your success:

They're the Best Bang for Your Hunger Buck: If you're reading this book, there's a good chance you're like me and you like to eat. Some (very few and lucky) people can eat a small bowl of soup for dinner and be done, and never think about food again until someone else reminds them it's mealtime. That would be nice, wouldn't it? Well, you can get pretty close to there too when you start to embrace veggies! As I said, I don't want you to get too wrapped up in calories, but metabolically, your body does work under the calorie system—using that energy from food and storing the excess as fat. Keeping this biological process in mind, if you're trying to feel satisfied without overdoing calories, it pays to eat foods that don't have a lot of calories but do make you feel full. That's exactly what veggies do. So whether you're talking celery or cauliflower, broccoli or beets, the "cost" is very low on them, calorically speaking, but the value is extremely high, volume and nutritionally speaking. When you fill up on veggies it makes it more likely your body will need to pull energy/calories from existing body fat (thus helping you burn fat) while still feeling satisfied. Nobody gains weight eating lots of vegetables, and as a matter of fact, the more veggies that you eat, the more weight you can lose.

The Fiber Has Real Effects on Hunger: For a long time, fiber was stereotyped as something that you only thought about if you had constipation. But the nutrient is more than just a nutritional way to help the digestive trains run on regular time; fiber has incredible health benefits as well (as it's linked to lower cholesterol and more). But when it comes to weight loss, the effect is crucial: Fiber is the barge of the digestive system, not the speed boat. That's a good thing, because the slower something moves through, the fuller you feel after eating it.

So when you add more of these fiber-rich vegetables, you're sending signals all through your body that you're not hungry, you don't need any pick-me-ups, you're perfectly fine, thank you very much. If it sounds too good to be true, try it. And take a minute now to think about the last time you had one too many sweets? Did you eat a lot of veggies in the meal beforehand?

Plant-Based Power Fortifies Your Whole Body: So much research revolves around the medicinal effects of vegetables, especially their ability to fight and prevent disease through a variety of vitamins, minerals and unique plant compounds known as phytonutrients. These micronutrients (which vary from veggie to veggie) have been linked to antioxidant properties. Let me explain what that term antioxidant is and why it has meaning. We are faced with free radical oxidation every day in the form of harmful toxins, from UV rays, pollution and the foods we eat. Think of your cells as a set of dominoes. When one cell is exposed to a free radical, it can cause a wave of oxidation and inflammation, connected to many highly preventable diseases like heart disease, diabetes, stroke and many cancers. Antioxidants stop oxidation, meaning they pick up the dominoes and prevent spillover. And while those might not be your immediate weight-loss goals, it does certainly speak to the power they have in terms of total-body health (especially considering that obesity is indeed related to and a risk factor for so many other diseases).

Veggies Help Improve Your Overall Gut Health: When I talk to people about their gut, they often think "gut" refers to a tiny hole or pouch in their stomach. The truth is that your "gut" is your entire digestive tract, from your tongue to your bum. This roller coaster takes your food on quite a ride—traveling through your body, twisting and turning, going up and down, and sometimes it throws you for a loop. During the process, the food that you chew slowly forms into your bowel movement. As it forms, the content of the stool is that food that ends up feeding microbes lining your bowel. These bacteria are either good (like lactobacillus) or bad (like *E. coli*), and the goal for having a good microbiome—the ecosystem of your bacteria—isn't just having only good bacteria. It's about having a ratio of more good than bad. To have a good ratio, you need a diverse colony.

Picture the bacteria as little bugs (they are alive, after all). If you give them food, they will grow, like a baby. The good bugs, probiotics, eat prebiotics. Prebiotics are the food that fuels these good bugs and helps them grow (and that's better for your health). What are prebiotics exactly? What do these good bugs like to eat? Vegetables. The fiber in vegetables. On the other hand, the bad bugs eat sugars. So if you eat a lot of processed and oily, sugary food, you'll tend to feed more bad bugs then good bugs. And they'll grow in numbers—and manipulate your cravings to make you want to eat more of those foods.

However, with the more veggies you eat, you create a stool that feeds your good gut bacteria—which can help with cravings, staving off obesity, promoting good digestive health, lowering stress and so much more.

So if you look at those four main points, there's really no reason not to load your plate with "Veggies Most." While I know veggies sometimes get a bad rap, I can excuse-proof them for you. Take a look:

If you think...
THEY'RE NOT EASY TO MAKE.

Then...
Bite-size raw veggies make great snacks. Cherry tomatoes, baby carrots, little cucumbers. They're easy to have on hand and will get you into the mode of reaching for the crunchiness (and even saltiness, depending on what you do to them) of veggies, rather than a processed snack. If you want delicious cooked recipes ready in minutes, see the recipes in Chapter 6.

If you think...

They make you gassy.

Then...

Take comfort in the fact that the fizz that comes from certain foods is because of the bacteria. The fizz happens because bacteria, when they eat fibers, ferment and give off CO_2 and other gases as an aftereffect. So when you're eating a lot of veggies and have gas, it's a good sign of a working digestive tract and healthy gut. Don't worry. That system becomes more efficient as time goes on.

If you think...

You don't like them.

Then...

The more you eat veggies, the more your body wants and craves them. You don't need to eat a million different varieties. You can start with two to three that you enjoy. As you drop pounds, you'll want to take on new ones, because the more veggie-based dishes you eat and grow accustomed to like, the more confident you will become that you will be able to sustain your weight loss.

If you think...

They taste bland.

Then...

Don't eat veggies naked—unless you want to! On 2B Mindset, you can add a little sugar, fat and salt (what I call Accessories, see page 116) to make them more appealing. If cheesy breadcrumbs over broccoli is helping you lose six pounds—because it's a lot better for you than cheesy nachos— then that's a good thing, because you're eating more and dropping weight. Same goes for dressings, which have been unfairly demonized by diet gurus: If you take some honey vinaigrette

The Right Hand vs. Left Hand Idea of Food

Many people look at weight loss as a short-term tactic. They will push through a short spurt of discipline in order to get results and don't care to think about what will happen next. It is very possible that you've done this at some point in your past. One of the ways you can lose this weight more easily—and ensure you lose it once and for all—is to get real with your mindset. The second you equate healthy foods with being a treat and not a chore, your weight loss will accelerate, and you'll be much more confident in your ability to keep the weight off for good.

Take out your two hands. Imagine your left hand as your "favorite" junk foods: cheesy pizza, gummy bears, donuts, cookies, whipped frozen coffee drinks, ice cream, bacon cheeseburgers, fries and chocolate—whatever you want.

On the right hand are meals filled with veggies and lean proteins that help you lose weight, like soups, stir-fries, salads, snackable veggies and dips, carrots and guacamole, roasted vegetables, protein shakes, omelets, grilled salmon and sauteed Brussels sprouts.

If the left hand is held high up on a pedestal, and looked at with longing eyes of "Ahh, I just wish I could eat that all day, I'm so in love with those foods," while the right hand is hanging down below your waist, relegated to being a chore and punishment, I hate to say it, but you'll never fully adopt the mindset and lose weight long term and keep it off.

If you see the left hand foods as ones you don't need and the right hand foods as necessary means for getting to your goals, you will have more success losing weight but still no guarantee for long-term success.

The only way to really drop this weight and keep it off (which you can see pretty clearly when you study adults who are at a healthy weight and maintain it) is to really glorify and uplift that right hand while getting clear on the negative results that the left hand has on your mind and body.

It's key to stop looking at that left hand as your lover. It's more of a nemesis or, better yet, something not even worth your time or energy. Rather than paint this positive picture of comfort and romance, you need to get clear of the struggles they lead you to. It's important to associate these foods with the feeling of not being in control, not feeling confident or energetic, feeling regretful or at a loss, and potentially even physically drained and uncomfortable. Once you start practicing Water First and Veggies Most, you know you feel better. You may see immediate changes to your skin, energy, digestion, and weight loss. You need to know it, and you need to own it. Veggies can't be something you eat because I or another health practitioner told you so—you need to feel a deep appreciation for the fact that they can taste good, fill you up, make you feel great, and get you dropping weight. Proteins need to be viewed as helping you stay full and in control, and help you make your physique more lean.

If you can practice this key aspect of cognitive behavioral therapy and reframe your mindset, weight loss will start to feel like a breeze. It doesn't come fast; it comes with practice and with the tracker and the scale. When you eat a ton of veggies, feel full, track it to be aware of it and see the positive change the next day on the scale, it will reinforce your new habits and you will continue to raise up that right hand with energy and gusto. It'll help form a habit and muscle memory for reaching for veggies more often as positive reinforcements, solidify veggies as your comfort food. And believe me, when you get to that point, which you may think is impossible now, weight loss will feel like the most effortless and enjoyable process of your life.

Similarly, when you do indulge in a food from your left hand, rather than deny it, you write about it in your tracker and see the impact it has on your energy and mood, and you will start to view it as beneath you; unworthy of your attention, time and energy.

When you explore the recipes in this program and start making the turnip fries and cauliflower rice risotto and fried rice, you'll wonder how that left hand ever had any leverage in the first place.

and chopped bacon and pour it over Brussels sprouts, suddenly you're eating more Brussels sprouts, a good thing. You only have an issue when you put sugar, salt and fat on more fat and silly carbs, like mayo on greasy fries, or candy bacon on a burger.

Besides the dozens of veggie-plus-accessories variations that I show you in this book, see my videos and the other resources within the 2B Mindset and The Mindset Membership for more ideas.

Ultimately, what you're going to be doing is redefining the way you think about veggies. If you've been hesitant to make them a big part of your diet, I am confident that you will learn to like them—and the many different ways that you can prepare them. And it won't be in an "I like them because I have to" kind of way, but an "I like them, really like them" kind of way.

My best source of veggie recipes has always been from my "naturally thin" friends who grew up in "naturally thin" homes that never focused on eating veggies as part of a diet. They have endless ideas of how to whip them up well based on years of eating them in their home, on their travels and in restaurants. I just asked one of these friends for the recipe for an asparagus salad she made, and do you know what it had in it? Agave, beer mustard, lemon juice, olive oil, salt and pepper. I've started making it regularly and, next thing you know, everyone in my family is gobbling up asparagus.

People think "veggies" means raw carrots and celery sticks. That's not what they have to be (unless, of course, you love those!). They can have sweet and salty flavors. One of my clients microwaves green beans from the bag then sautés them in a pan with slivered almonds and Everything But The Bagel seasoning. She feasts on them and is still losing pounds. As I said, nobody is gaining weight eating vegetables.

FOOD LISTS

TO VIEW THE FULL LISTS (AND THE UK FOOD LISTS) FOR EACH FOOD GROUP,
CHECK OUT THE "RESOURCES" SECTION ON THE 2B MINDSET PROGRAM PAGE.

🧂 *When you see this icon next to a food, it is a reminder that it can be high in sodium.*

Veggies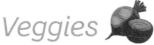

PURPOSE: To make you full! We always want veggies to be our first bite, and they should make up most of our lunch and dinner plates!

- Artichokes
- Arugula
- Asparagus
- Beet greens
- Beets
- Bok choy
- Broccoli
- Broccolini
- Broccoli slaw
- Brussels sprouts
- Butterhead lettuce
- Button mushrooms
- Cabbage (all varieties)
- Cactus
- Carrots (all varieties)
- Cauliflower/ cauliflower rice
- Celery
- Celery root
- Chanterelle mushrooms
- Chayote
- Chinese cabbage
- Collard greens
- Cremini mushrooms
- Cucumbers (all varieties)
- Dandelion greens
- Eggplant

- Endive
- Enoki mushrooms
- Fennel
- Green beans
- Green bell pepper
- Hearts of palm
- Jerusalem artichoke
- Jicama
- Kale
- Kohlrabi
- Leek
- Mesclun
- Morel mushrooms
- Mustard greens
- Napa cabbage
- Okra
- Onions (all varieties)
- Orange bell pepper
- Oyster mushrooms
- 🧂 Pickled and fermented veggies (kimchi, sauerkraut, etc.)
- 🧂 Pickles
- Porcini mushrooms
- Portobello mushrooms
- Radicchio
- Radishes/daikon

- Rainbow chard
- Rapini (broccoli rabe)
- Red bell pepper
- Rhubarb
- Romaine lettuce
- Seaweed, raw
- Shakeology Boost: Power Greens*
- Shallots
- Shiitake mushrooms
- Snow peas
- Spaghetti squash
- Spinach
- Sprouts
- String beans
- Sugar snap peas
- Summer squash
- Swiss chard
- Tomatillos
- Tomatoes (all varieties)
- Turnip
- Turnip greens
- Water chestnuts
- Watercress
- Yellow bell pepper
- Yellow squash
- Zucchini

*All products and flavors may not be available in your market.

Taste the Rainbow!

Colorful veggies and fruit are abundant with nutrients!

RED in veggies and fruits means that they contain lycopene! These antioxidants can help promote heart health! So... include red fruits and vegetables, like tomatoes, in your mix to boost the nutritional value of your meals!

Keep those eyes sparkling by filling your meals with **ORANGE** fruits and veggies. Beta-carotene, abundant in orange produce, is a powerful antioxidant, which can be converted into vitamin A. These orange additions, like carrots, aid in improving eye health, benefiting your immune system, as well as preventing skin damage. Win-win-win!!!

YELLOW/WHITE veggies and fruits are high in antioxidants such as vitamin C! Chop up and mix in those yellows, like onion, turnip and garlic, to improve heart health, enhance your immune system and promote eye health!

GO GREEN! These veggies and fruits are abundant in vitamins, minerals, phytochemicals and fiber!!! Greens are especially rich in vitamin K and B vitamins, which act to improve heart health, protect bones, and so much more! Consume these low-calorie, fiber-rich veggies, like spinach, brussels sprouts, and sugar snap peas to keep you nourished from head to toe!

FEELING PURPLE/BLUE?! Anthocyanins, an antioxidant in purplish-blue veggies and fruit, like red cabbage and eggplant, give them their color! They are healthy for your heart. In herbal medicine, these colorful goodies are used to promote a healthy urinary tract. (We have lots of great and unexpected recipes in Chapter 6 for this category!)

PROTEIN: **HAVE IT AT EVERY MEAL**
Why: *It Helps Keep You Full and Satisfied*

I N MY MIND, I think of veggies as the kings of nutrition. They have the power. They rule how your body operates. And they have a long (and scientifically supported) tradition of nutritional majesty.

When I think about proteins, I have to put them in my royal family as well, like the queen, essential for ruling your body in the right way (or something like that). That's because they, too, have so much nutritional influence over how your body operates, and your overall sense of control around food.

While some people have a good idea about what protein is—yes, it's found prominently in meat and chicken, but it's also in other foods, like cheese, eggs, shrimp, smoked salmon, sausages, tofu, beans, Shakeology, BEACHBARS—not everybody understands its role. Some people associate protein with muscle-building—i.e., if you have a lot of protein, your muscles are going to bulk up to the size of small cars. Protein is a building block for muscles, but it's not true that eating protein will muscle you up to sizes you don't want.

In fact, the opposite is true: Protein can help slim you down while maintaining a lean physique.

In your body, protein gets broken down into amino acids, which are indeed important building blocks for cells in your body. The main reason why I like proteins is that they go a long way in helping you feel satiated—which certainly is one of the key components to curbing hunger and cravings throughout the day. So if you make sure to get enough protein, then you can really fend off hunger pangs and cravings—enemy number one for people who want to lose weight.

To make your protein intake work best, I recommend these four tactics become part of your daily eating approach:

Ilana-ism

Measure Your Proteins, Measure Your Progress

It's easier to gauge how satisfied you are and how you feel if you eat
trackable proteins. For example, take chicken on the bone.
You can write in "2 chicken thighs" or "1 drumstick"on your tracker and
have a better understanding about how much protein you've eaten
and how you feel afterward. Eggs are another good example.
Was it two eggs or three eggs that helped me stay full and satisfied?
This is in contrast to ground beef or stir-fries that can leave you guessing.
1 Fist = apx. 1 cup to help you eyeball it and track with more detail.

Have protein at every meal: You'll find my complete list of protein
sources on page 105, so you'll know you have plenty of options to eat at
every meal. Many people don't find it difficult to have protein for dinner, but lunch and breakfast are more difficult for some people. That's
for a number of reasons: One, we've long been conditioned that appropriate breakfast foods are cereal and toast, and a sandwich and chips
for lunch. Two, in our hectic days, we often skip breakfast or choose
grab-and-go options, which are usually handheld items, like muffins,
bagels and carby snacks. And as for lunch, sandwiches, even when they
contain protein in the center, are usually mainly carbs as well, especially when they are made with a thick loaf of ciabatta and a default bag
of chips on the side.

But even your breakfast should include a protein source, which
could come from eggs (hard-boiled are easy to eat on the run) or a protein shake, like Shakeology. And you don't have to rule out traditional
dinner-type proteins either, as grilled steak that's saved and heated up
can make a nice breakfast option, too. No matter what you choose, your
goal is to get some protein at every meal. It will help you feel full, and it

will take up space that you might otherwise fill with sugary options—
which would cause spikes in energy and make you hungry very soon
after you eat it. How much protein? While I won't have you weighing
ounces, you'll see how to understand how much is too much or too little
later in this chapter.

Pick your favorites as go-tos: You could pick a lot of words or phrases
that justify our obesity epidemic: comfort food, processed food, all-you-
can-eat buffets, value meals, bottomless mimosas, unlimited bread-
sticks . . .the list is endless. But here's one that I think is a major con-
tributor: convenience. While eating (and emotions and circumstances
that surround eating) are complicated, it is true that our busy lives have
steered us to make decisions based on convenience over health. And
many times, it's not convenient to have protein—or at least it doesn't feel
like it. Eat a cookie or make a Shakeology? Grill a piece of meat or order
a pizza? Whip up an omelet or hit the drive-through? We know which
ones seem easier to do—at least at first glance. So the way to attack this
is head-on. You have to *make* it convenient to eat your protein. That can
come in the form of always having hard-boiled eggs or turkey slices on
hand, grilling up chicken and saving it for the week, prepping a bean dish
that's ready to go, or keeping string cheese and Greek yogurt stocked in
your fridge. You can also keep jerky or BEACHBARS in your office or car
to ensure you have a smart protein fix when you want a filling snack and
all that's around are pretzels and candied nuts. Whatever your favorite
form of protein is, find a way to make it easy to eat—and then you will.

Mix them up: Part of the reason I love protein sources is that they
pair beautifully with veggies. Think about all the options you have—
veggie omelette, chicken fajitas, salmon salads, beef and broccoli, and
so many more. I also love sneaking veggies into a smoothie, like mix-

ing chocolate Shakeology with frozen cauliflower rice, nut butter, and almond milk for a delicious (and easy to make on-the-go) shake. The point is that there are so many different ways to consume protein that you don't have to feel limited by just a few options.

In a pinch, default to protein: One of the main points about the 2B Mindset is that you do have the flexibility to live your life—and enjoy it. No matter where the party is happening, no matter how plans change, no matter what life throws your way, it's typically not too hard to make protein a part of every meal or social situation.

Eating out? You can usually order a chicken/fish/meat with two sides of vegetables anywhere you go. You can go with sashimi, edamame, a cucumber salad and a seaweed salad at a sushi place, or chicken and vegetables at Asian restaurants. How about meatballs and a Caesar salad at an Italian place? Even at parties, you can load up on the veggie tray, as well as some shrimp cocktail or chicken skewers.

What are BEACHBARS?

As you may realize, I am a serious chocolate lover.
One of my favorite ways to get my chocolate fix is Beachbody
BEACHBARS. These on-the-go snack bars have only 150 calories
with 9–10 grams of protein and 4 g of fiber, which helps keep you
satisfied longer. The best part is that they are individually wrapped
so you can indulge your sweet craving while staying in control.

PROTEINS

PURPOSE: To help keep you fuller longer, so be sure to enjoy some at every meal.

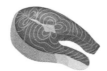

EGGS AND DAIRY

- Cheese, all varieties and flavors (light, low-fat, or reduced-fat)
- Cottage cheese (1–2%)
- Egg whites
- Eggs, whole
- Greek yogurt (plain, 0–2%)
- Ricotta cheese (part-skim)
- Yogurt (plain, 1–2%)

CHICKEN AND TURKEY

- Chicken or turkey breast, skinless, boneless; or on-the-bone
- Chicken or turkey deli slices (nitrite-free)
- Chicken or turkey drumsticks, skinless
- Chicken or turkey thighs, skinless, boneless; or on-the-bone
- Ground chicken or turkey (≤ 93% lean)

BEEF AND PORK

- Beef chuck shoulder steak
- Beef top round (steak and roast)
- Beef top sirloin steak
- Ground beef (≤ 95% lean)
- Ham slices (nitrite-free)
- Pork tenderloin

SEAFOOD

- Clams
- Cod
- Crab
- Halibut
- Lobster
- Octopus
- Oysters
- Salmon
- Sashimi/raw fish/sushi (wrapped in cucumber or seaweed instead of rice)
- Scallops
- Shrimp
- Sole
- Tilapia
- Tuna (canned or in pouch; light or white in water)

shakeology*

- Café Latte
- Café Latte Vegan
- Chocolate
- Chocolate Vegan
- Greenberry
- Strawberry
- Tropical Strawberry Vegan
- Vanilla
- Vanilla Vegan

DAILY SUNSHINE*

- Chocolate
- Strawberry Banana

BEACHBAR

- Chocolate Cherry Almond
- Peanut Butter Chocolate
- Plant-Based Chocolate Almond Crunch

PLANT-BASED PROTEIN

- Edamame (organic)
- Lupini beans
- Protein powder (hemp, pea, quinoa, rice)
- Seitan
- Soybeans (organic)
- Tempeh (organic)
- Tofu (organic, extra firm)
- Vegan Shakeology, 1 scoop
- Veggie burger (with at least 10 g protein)

Tip If you're short on time or aren't the cooking kind, you can find many protein options packaged and ready to eat, along with pre-cooked and frozen options, so you can easily pull together a meal in minutes.

*All products and flavors may not be available in your market.

CARBOHYDRATES (FFCS):
KEEP SERVINGS UNDER 150 CALORIES
Why: They Give You Energy

YOU THINK POLITICS and sports are the big pot-stirrers during dinner-table discussions? Try saying the word "carbs" among people who deal with food, health and bodies for a living. In these circles, carbohydrates have spurred more debate than just about any nutritional hot-button issue that I can remember.

There's a group that classifies carbs as pure evil. They see it as a macronutrient that they have no control of. They think it works like an instant injection of fat into your body and they beat themselves up when they "cheat." Then there's another group that thinks this is way too extreme of a position—that carbs are part of a holistic approach to eating. My view of carbs is found somewhere in the middle: They certainly don't need to be banned, but they should be controlled.

There's good reason for that: Carbs are made of sugars, starches and fiber. The fiber component to carbohydrates will keep you full and in more control of your food. Fibrous foods also tend to contain a lot of other nutrients. Since fiber is structural, the fiber is typically concentrated in the exterior layer of the food—like the peel or skin of an apple, potatoes and beans, and the brown/bran layer of grains.

Starches, even ones that don't taste too sweet, like rice and bread, also break down into sugars in the body. These sugars become a primary source of energy. They help fuel your systems, including your brain. They help you feel more energetic, and they can provide a long-lasting source of power for your body.

I say that with a note of caution, however, because the quality and quantity of carbs matter. Most carbohydrates found in nature—beans, fruits, whole grains—contain fiber. Fiber works as the bodyguard to ensure that you are never taking in too much sugar without the help of fiber to slow its release into your bloodstream. I break down carbs into two categories: fiber-filled carbs, aka "FFCs," and "silly carbs."

FFCs

Carbohydrates filled with fiber, FFCs, take longer for your body to break down and digest, which is why they are sometimes referred to as "complex." That complexity is a good thing and provides a slow drip of energy that your organs and systems need to operate most efficiently. Examples like starchy veggies, beans and legumes, and whole grains are good for your body, providing a slow and steady supply of energy that our body can burn off.

To help you visualize them: Imagine a zoomed-in picture of a piece of whole wheat or wild rice. The outer layer is the bran, the complex part that's made up of fiber. Next is the center of the whole grain, the endosperm. That's the sugary, starchy center. Finally, there's a small aspect of a whole grain called the germ, which contains healthy fats and other nutrients.

We want that bran layer always attached to the endosperm because that slows down our ability to break down that sugary, starchy center. That way, we have more stable blood sugar levels and energy going forward. This is also much better for overall weight loss.

FFCs are helpful for a couple reasons: One, they have the full-feeling benefits of fiber. Two, they help you avoid the crash-and-burn-and-eat affect that simple carbs can have.

Silly Carbs

When carbs are stripped of their fiber through processing, as in white bread, pasta, crackers, candy and cake, the body absorbs the sugar more rapidly. This causes our blood sugar levels to rise (unnaturally), forcing our body to produce excess insulin to regulate it. I call these carbs "silly carbs" because it's fine to be silly on occasion, and you certainly can enjoy some along your weight loss, but you'll want to be "smarter" more often for more successful results. (And FYI, insulin is a fat-storing hormone, so these foods cause quick weight gain as well.)

We often turn to silly carbs because they provide that quick boost of energy (or comfort) that's extra appealing when we're feeling sluggish. Unfortunately, that extreme spike leads to an extreme drop, causing you to feel tired and want another boost. So what do you do to get that pickup? Reach for more instant energy. But because your body can't process it all, that eventually leads to more fat storage, and you wanting even more. It's a vicious silly carb cycle.

Health issues aside, these fiberless carbs are an issue because they increase appetite and promote further cravings. You don't have to ban them—believe me, I certainly don't—but you will have to track them (yes, every one of them) and prioritize your favorite indulgences for special occasions.

Ultimately, you'll want to do this anyway, because through daily weigh-ins, you will see the effect they have on your weight. With tracking, you'll discover the impact that they have on your behaviors so you can achieve better self-control around food. When you eat them in the order of my More? Sure! Model (see Chapter 7), you will see how these silly treats fit in with the 2B Mindset and your weight loss.

So to break that cycle without sacrificing the energy you need, use the following guidelines to help you decipher whether it's a silly carb or an FFC.

Choose ones you won't overeat: A lot of weight-loss success revolves around nutrition, but I have seen firsthand how much environment, emotions and your past habits play a role in what and how you eat. If every time you bring home that baguette, you can't stop eating it, then why bring it home again? Some brands are upfront with the addictive nature of their foods. Pringles' slogan is literally "Once you pop, you can't stop."

Be aware of "open-ended foods," a term I coined for things like that large bag of tortilla chips or pretzels sitting in your pantry. There are 12 servings per bag—how many do you think you've eaten at a time? If carbs have been your weakness, and you have a history of overeating them, then you will want to choose carbs with a clear and realistic end or serving size. I recommend sticking to trackable carbs like whole pieces of fruit, 100-calorie bags of popcorn or bean snacks, and pre-sliced bread. When you create an environment where the best foods for your weight loss are readily available, it's much easier to make good choices. But if you have an environment where your pantry is filled with not-so-good tongue-tempters, you're going to have a much harder time. So step one is focusing on foods that you won't overeat. I'm not saying you should pick ones that you don't like at all, but choose ones that you're less likely to gorge on.

Ilana-ism

Open-Ended Foods

Large, seemingly bottomless containers of silly carbs. Examples include a bag of chips, a tub of cheese balls or three rows of sandwich cookies. Stick to FFCs you can track.

Choose ones with about 150 calories or less per serving, and know how many servings there are: Here's where label reading comes in handy. Sometimes you will see a bran muffin listed as 180 calories per serving, but there are *two* servings in the single muffin. *Pass*. When one serving of carbs has more than 150 calories in it, it usually has unnecessary added sugars and fats as well. Try to stick to one portion at a meal as well, and use the Plate It! instructions (see later in this chapter) and More? Sure! Model to guide you. If you're more active, or would like an additional serving of carbohydrates, be sure to track it in detail so you can see how it's working for you.

HOW TO READ A NUTRITION LABEL

Sugary Cereal

Nutrition Facts

Servings per container about 9
Serving size   **1 cup (32g)**

Amount per serving

Calories   130

Total Fat	1.5 g
Saturated Fat	0 g
Trans Fat	0 g
Polyunsaturated Fat	0.5 g
Monounsaturated Fat	1 g
Cholesterol	0 mg
Sodium	160 mg
Potassium	50 mg
Total Carbohydrate	27 g
Dietary Fiber	1 g
Total Sugars	10 g
Other Carbohydrate	16 g
Protein	1 g

Ingredients: Whole Grain Corn, Sugar, Corn Meal, Corn Syrup, Rice Bran and/or Canola Oil, Salt, Color (vegetable and fruit juice, turmeric extract and annatto extract), Trisodium Phosphate, Natural Flavor, Citric Acid, Malic Acid.

Bran Flake Cereal

Nutrition Facts

About 10 servings per container
Serving size   **1 cup**

Amount per serving

Calories   130

Total Fat	1 g
Saturated Fat	0 g
Trans Fat	0 g
Polyunsaturated Fat	0 g
Monounsaturated Fat	0 g
Cholesterol	0 mg
Sodium	125 mg
Total Carbohydrate	32 g
Dietary Fiber	7 g
Total Sugars	3 g
Protein	5 g

Ingredients: Organic Whole Grain Wheat, Organic Wheat Bran, Organic Cane Sugar, Organic Barley Malt Extract, Sea Salt.

SILLY CARBS. No thanks!

FFCs! Yum!

Ilana-ism

An Open Face Is a Happy Face

You'll begin to feel the benefits of keeping your protein portion at least the same (if not greater) than your portion of carbs. When you analyze a typical American meal starring a burger, it's surrounded in carbs, with two hunks of bread per one patty, plus a pile of fries, and usually a soda or shake. Same goes for a sandwich and chips. One way to even out the ratios and have them work better for you and your weight loss is to remove the top bun. That way, you have one burger patty to one piece of the bun, making the protein-to-carb ratio more balanced. However, the buns served at most restaurants are white bread, making them a silly carb. So, to make a smarter choice, skip the bun altogether and ask for your burger in a lettuce wrap or on a bed of lettuce and enjoy it with an FFC like a small side of sweet potato wedges or a bean-based soup.

Side note: You will redefine the meaning of 'it's sooo good," because with your weight loss goal bright in mind, you will see that to be "really good" you'll want it to taste good but also be good for your weight loss.

So let's deflate the notion that all carbs are bad—and really think about what kind of energy source they can be and how they can positively support your weight loss.

Get at least 1 gram of fiber for every 10 grams of total carbs: The more fiber, the better! There are so many claims and marketing tactics on the front of a product; flip the food around for the actual facts. While you're label-stalking, inspect how many grams of fiber the food contains. Compare that to the total carbs—so if the label shows 30 grams of total carbs, you want at least 3 grams of fiber. That ensures the food has fiber in a healthy ratio. While you're at it, check the grams of sugar. Ideally the food has more fiber grams than sugar grams in it, or close to that. The more fiber and the less sugar, the better your ability to control your consumption and lose weight with it. This tactic will help you save so much money and clear up confusion next time you're food shopping.

Great examples of FFCs are foods like beans, plain oatmeal and berries. They're foods that have been shown to have health benefits, including promoting heart health. And they're foods that will help you with weight loss because they—in combination with your veggies and protein—will give you sustained energy throughout the day.

As I've said, I don't want you to worry about counting nutrients or going crazy trying to figure out calculations of foods. These recommendations aren't even necessarily coming from the perspective of a dietitian, but from someone who ate Oreos and Girl Scout cookies a sleeve at a time. I am now able to have one cookie, really enjoy it and stop. You will get there, too. It will take practice, but even if you have a sweet tooth or are a self-proclaimed "carboholic," you will be able to drop weight without dropping carbs.

I want you to help stave off hunger with smart food choices. And I want you to eat the foods that will help you see the number on the scale go down. When it comes to carbs, you need the knowledge to make smart choices. Eventually, the practice of identifying the FFCs and reducing silly carbs will become second nature.

"Is fruit really a carb?" I say Veggies Most a lot, so a common question that comes up is: What about fruit? Well, fruit is a carb, and when I started realizing that, about 20 pounds down along my weight-loss journey, I was able to seriously start dropping sizes. While we have always been told to eat lots of fruits and veggies, when it comes to weight loss, you still need to be eating Veggies Most, because fruit functions as a carbohydrate. It is much more similar calorically and nutritionally to a slice of whole wheat bread than it is to a cucumber.

Take a medium apple, a slice of bread and about a cup of cucumber slices. The medium apple and the slice of bread both contain about 90 to 95 calories, and have about 20 grams of carbohydrates (and about 4 to 5 grams of fiber). Nutritionally, they're a lot more similar than they are to a cup of cucumbers, which has closer to 15 calories, and 3 to 4 grams of carbohydrates. You can and should enjoy nature's candy, but be sure to track it and see how it works for you best. (For a breakdown of the lowest sugar and most trackable fruits, watch the Carbohydrates video at 2BMindset.com.)

CARBOHYDRATES / FFCS

PURPOSE: To give you energy. Fiber-Filled Carbohydrates (aka FFCs) are the kind we will focus on—because the fiber in carbs makes the energy last longer and they're better for weight loss.

STARCHY VEGGIES
- Acorn squash
- Butternut squash
- Corn
- Green peas
- Plantains
- Potato
- Sweet potato

BEANS AND LEGUMES

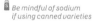
Be mindful of sodium if using canned varieties

- Bean-based soup
- Bean pasta
- Beans, all varieties (black, cannellini, garbanzo, pinto, etc.)
- Hummus
- Lentils (black, brown, red)
- Peas (black-eyed, cow, etc.)

FRUITS
- Apples
- Banana
- Blackberries
- Blueberries
- Cantaloupe
- Grapefruit
- Grapes
- Honeydew melon
- Kiwifruit
- Mango
- Orange
- Peach
- Pear
- Pineapple
- Plum
- Raspberries
- Strawberries
- Watermelon

WHOLE GRAINS
- Barley
- Bran cereal* (low-sugar)
- Bread* (whole-grain)
- Crackers* (whole-grain)
- English muffin* (whole-grain)
- Oats (plain steel-cut, rolled, or instant with low- or no-added sugar)
- Pasta* (whole-grain)
- Pita bread* (whole-grain)
- Popcorn (with 0 g trans fats)
- Quinoa
- Sandwich slim* (whole-grain)
- Tortilla* (whole-grain)
- Waffles* (whole-grain)
- Wheat farina

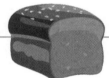

*CHECKLIST FOR BUYING FFCS:
→ Choose ones you won't overeat
→ The serving size is easy to track
→ It's 150 calories or less
→ There's at least 1 g fiber for every 10 g total carbs (but the more fiber, the better!)
→ Pick ones with the same, if not more, fiber grams than sugar grams
→ Pick ones without any trans fats (i.e., partially hydrogenated oil)

"SILLY" CARBS & TREATS

THESE ARE FOODS THAT:

- Are more indulgent
- Are harder to control
- Have little to no fiber, contain more grams of sugar and/or fat than fiber

Many "silly" carbs and treats cause energy spikes and dives. They aren't the smartest for your weight loss or mindset. It's okay to be silly on occasion, but try to prioritize your favorite sweets and treats—a little silliness here and there isn't a problem, as long as you track it. But ultimately, making smarter and stronger choices will make your weight loss smarter and stronger.

- Alcohol
  (beer, liquor, wine)
- Baked goods, all varieties
  (brownies, cakes, cookies, donuts, etc.)
- Candy and chocolates, all varieties
- Chips, all varieties
- Coffee creamer
- Deep-fried foods
  (Battered/fried chicken or fish,
  French fries, tater tots, etc.)
- Frozen treats
  (ice cream, ice pops,
  yogurt, or comparable
  non-dairy frozen treat)
- Sugar-sweetened beverages
  (juices, lemonades, teas, etc.)

Tips If you have it, track it. You'll be surprised that a sweet or treat on occasion won't cause such a big weight gain. So savor it, enjoy it and own it by writing it down in your tracker and going on the scale the next day. You will start to learn what is most worth it to you.

It's usually easier to enjoy it and track it later when it's something you can measure or remember, like 1 cookie or square of chocolate versus "handfuls of chips," which can leave you questioning what may have caused the scale to go up.

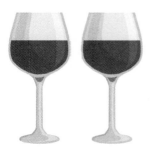

ACCESSORIES: USE THEM, EAT THEM, LOVE THEM!
Why: They Help You Eat More Veggies and Make Meals Pop with Flavor

WHEN YOU THINK of "accessories," you may picture a cool pair of shades, a hot pair of shoes for your night-out outfit, a fun case for your phone or a snappy hat for your beach vacation.

Their supporting role is clear: They may not be the main feature, but they sure do make things a whole lot more fun. They enhance the look and feel of the outfit, and in some cases, add a useful function as well.

When it comes to nutrition, my "accessories" do the same thing. They have a supporting job—and that is to make your meals and your food pop with flavor, to turn something that could be bland into something that's, well, just awesome. I am obsessed with flavor and am always on the hunt for finding ways to make my meals elevated and more delicious. For me, food can't just be "fuel," it has to be satisfying. And in my study of my clients and their success, it is proven that sugar, salt and fat make food more delicious, enjoyable and, in fact, a little addictive. Can you imagine how good you would look and feel if you used those adjectives to describe veggies? Guess what? You can. While there are too many causes of the obesity crisis to point fingers at just one, I truly blame anyone who has publicly shamed salad dressings and toppings as a real cause. In my experience losing 100 pounds while maintaining a love for volume, food and flavor, I can tell you that no one ever gains weight from eating a reasonable amount of salad dressing on their salads.

In fact, it wasn't until I figured this out that I was able to truly believe I could lose weight and get the motivation I needed to start. As a kid with parents who were constantly dieting, I distinctly remember being told: "Ilana, if it tastes good, it can't be good for you." This sabotaged my efforts, because my only choices presented were obesity or misery—and that's simply not the reality. You can get slim while still getting great pleasure from the flavors you love. Tasty food can be some of the best food for you!

These accessories may have more fat and sugar, but you're using them sparingly as a way to help you to eat and enjoy more veggies. And that's the perfect way to think about them. You're not going to lose weight if you slurp down a bowl of fondue or pour that cheese all over a stuffed potato or bread bowl, but you will if you drizzle some over a mound of broccoli. You're not going to lose weight if you wolf down a box of sugary cereal, but you will if you sprinkle a little sugar and cinnamon on a big bowl of spaghetti squash for a sweet and savory dish. And you're not going to lose weight with a bucket of beach fries, but you will if you coat some roasted cauliflower with salt, garlic and olive oil and dip it in a lightened-up ranch dressing. And in the end—because you're using accessories well—you won't have to sacrifice taste or flavor (or feel like you're denying your cravings).

Sure, you will want to be savvy about your accessories, like my diluting technique below, but you will never deprive yourself of them. A main factor why my "bunnies" keep their weight off is because they're satisfied, not deprived, along the way. If you feel like you need to go gorge on your "last meal" because you're about to embark on a four-month journey of steamed chicken breast and spinach, then think again. The2B Mindset helps you reframe your approach to flavor, dressings, condiments and sauces, so that you don't have to think of them as bad or off-limits. Rather, they are a necessary tool not only for losing weight happily, but certainly for keeping it off.

I'm certain that accessories will be one of your favorite allies in your approach to weight loss because you'll be able to experiment with all

ACCESSORIES

PURPOSE: To get you eating more veggies and make your meals pop with flavor!

GUIDELINES WHEN ENJOYING ACCESSORIES: Pick 1 or 2 per meal that you enjoy most. Start with less. If you want more, you can always add a little bit more later. And make sure to quantify them somehow so you can track them later. Whether you use a tablespoon or bottle cap, or compare them to a golf ball, you just want to keep your eye on them so you can track them.

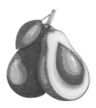

FATS

- Avocado and guacamole
- 🗋 Bacon, pork
- Butter
- Coconut milk (canned)
- 🗋 Full-fat cheese (blue, cheddar, feta, parmesan, pepper jack, etc.)
- 🗋 Natural nut butters (almond, cashew, peanut, etc.)
- 🗋 Nuts, whole and chopped
- Oil (avocado, grapeseed, olive, toasted sesame, etc.)
- 🗋 Olives
- Pesto
- 🗋 Sausage
- 🗋 Seeds (chia, flax, hemp, pumpkin, sesame, sunflower, etc.), whole, chopped, ground
- Sunflower seed butter (natural)

SUGARS

- Agave
- Brown sugar
- Dried fruit
- Honey
- Jelly and jams, all varieties
- Maple syrup

CONDIMENTS, DRESSINGS, SAUCES, AND MARINADES

🗋 *Be mindful of sodium in all of these items*

- Alfredo sauce
- Barbecue sauce
- Ketchup (without high-fructose corn syrup)
- Marinara sauce
- Mayonnaise (light or low-fat)
- Powdered peanut butter
- Salad dressings, all varieties (blue cheese, Italian, ranch, etc.)
- Sour cream (light or reduced-fat)
- Tomato paste
- Tomato sauce
- Vinaigrettes (balsamic, red wine, etc.)

BEVERAGES

Great for adding some to tea, coffee or your Shakeology but recommend having no more than 1 cup per day

- Milk (reduced-fat, 1–2%)
- Unsweetened plant-based milks (almond, cashew, organic soy, rice, etc.)

SHAKEOLOGY BOOSTS*

- Digestive Health
- Focused Energy

"FREEBIE" ACCESSORIES AND BEVERAGES

You can eat all you want of these accessories!

- 🗋 Broth (beef, chicken, fish and vegetable)
- Cocoa (cacao) powder
- Coffee, black, unsweetened
- Herbs, fresh, dried or frozen (basil, cilantro, dill, garlic, ginger, parsley, etc.)
- Horseradish
- Hot sauce
- Lemon juice
- Lime juice
- Monk fruit sweetener

ACCESSORIES

CHECKLIST FOR BUYING ACCESSORIES:

- Has 0–40 calories per Tbsp. or under 80 calories per 2 Tbsp.
- Ideally does not contain salt or sugar in the first two ingredients
- Has simple ingredients that don't contain artificial sugars, like sucralose, aspartame, Ace K, and are free of high-fructose corn syrup

"FREEBIES" CON'T.

- Mustard
- Salsa
- Seasoning blends (without salt or sugar in the first two ingredients)
- Seltzer water

- Soy sauce (reduced-sodium)
- Spices (cinnamon, cumin, pepper, turmeric, etc.)
- Stevia
- Tea, unsweetened
- Vinegar, unsweetened (apple cider, balsamic, red wine, rice wine, white, etc.)
- Water (of course!)

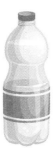

WATER BOOSTERS

- Aloe vera juice
- Cucumber
- Lemon
- Lime
- Mint
- Water enhancers (all-natural flavors)
- Whole fruit pieces (berries, mango, watermelon, etc.)

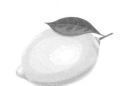

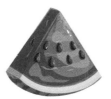

Tip If you want to enjoy an accessory (like a salad dressing or marinade) that has more than 40 calories per Tbsp., dilute 1 Tbsp. worth with 1 Tbsp. of water, vinegar, lemon or lime juice to help spread the flavor across the whole dish!

*All products and flavors may not be available in your market.

kinds of flavors to make your veggies (and proteins) taste absolutely delicious! Think of the possibilities with onion and garlic salt, guacamole, pesto, barbecue sauce, bacon and so many more.

I think my favorite part about accessories is that just a little bit can go a long way. You don't need gobs and gobs of sauces and dips to add flavor; you can simply start with a small amount and then add a little more at a time if you feel like you need it.

Here's my recommendation for how you can approach your accessories:

- When shopping for bottled, jarred and store-bought accessories, look at the nutritional label. If something has more grams of fat or sugar than anything else, then consider it an accessory.

- When thinking about calories, stick to things that have 40 calories or fewer per tablespoon or 80 calories per 2 tablespoons. And if you can keep your accessory under the 80 calories, that's a win, especially if you're using it for a mighty portion of veggies.

- Ideally, the first two ingredients aren't salt or sugar (it's okay if they're farther down the list).

- Choose ones that have simple ingredients and that don't contain artificial ingredients, like sucralose, aspartame or Ace K. They should also be free of high-fructose corn syrup.

Best of all, my list of accessories includes many "freebies" that you can use (or drink) as liberally as you want.

What About Fat?

Now that you've seen my approach to food groups and how to eat, you may be wondering what happened to dietary fat. After all, you probably have friends who talk nonstop about their experience with keto and all they can talk about is fat, fat, fat to lose fat, fat, fat.

Dietary fat does come in a variety of forms—unsaturated, saturated and trans. Unsaturated fats are the ones that are touted as the healthiest forms, as they are linked to many health benefits, including increased satiety and heart health. (Trans fats, found in processed foods, are the ones you want to avoid.)

I don't emphasize eating a certain amount of fat, because what I have seen over and over is that focusing on Veggies Most, protein at every meal, supplementary carbs and accessories as needed are the keys to successful and long-term weight loss. And here's the thing: With this way of eating, you will likely be getting more than enough fats in your diet. That's because most foods, as I said, are made up of a combination of various macronutrients. So if you're eating fish as your protein, you'll also be getting healthy fats in those servings. And you can also get healthy fats by drizzling extra virgin olive oil (an accessory) on your veggies and protein. Many of the foods in my accessories list—butter, sausage, avocado, nuts and nut butters—are high in fat.

My approach to fats is that you will get just enough of them, but because they are so calorie-dense, they should not be a main focus of how you eat. Fill that plate with veggies, protein and some FFCs, and you'll put yourself in great shape to get into, well, great shape.

What If I'm a Picky Eater?

Depending on how you grew up or what your diet has looked like lately, you may turn your nose up at veggies. *I just can't!* You can. Being a picky eater is okay; you just have to learn to overcome the fear of trying new veggies and apply what you like to what you want to eat. For starters, you have to be more open-minded and understand that our taste buds are always changing. What influences us and our habits and behaviors are always changing and evolving, too. Just because you didn't like these certain steamed, sad-looking or ill-prepared veggies as a kid does not mean you're not going to like them now. If you are a pizza lover but think you can't eat veggies, then you need to try adding a good marinara sauce and cheese to some roasted zucchini or check out the Zucchini Pizza Coins later in the book. Some of my favorite tips:

- *Go to a restaurant you already love.* If you love how they grill their steak or make their pizza, you'll probably like their heirloom tomato and burrata. And sautéed mushrooms. So go to a restaurant you already enjoy and just start playing with their sides. You could ask the waiter how they're made and then start infusing those cooking methods and veggies into your meals at home.

- *Mix them into your favorites.* If you love store-bought mac and cheese, I recommend just getting a bag of frozen broccoli florets, defrosting them and stirring them into the mac and cheese. You get all that flavor you love and now all of a sudden, you're eating a lot more broccoli, and you really can't even tell the difference. You could also just make the cheese sauce and swap the pasta for the broccoli. This will get you into the direction of being more open-minded that broccoli can taste flavorful when you do different things to it.

- ***Make sneaky substitutes.*** Let's take lasagna. If your current recipe layers meat sauce or ricotta cheese mixture and noodles plus tomato sauce, just slip in a nice layer of thinly sliced eggplant or zucchini. You probably won't even realize that it's there, but you and your family and everyone around you will be eating more veggies. Also, it's a subtle way to help them embrace veggie textures and flavors and all the nutrition that they can offer you.

  Or let's say you like meatballs and rice. You'll probably like meatballs and cauliflower rice. If you like pasta with vodka sauce, try mixing the sauce with zucchini noodles.

- ***When in doubt, stir-fry.*** You don't have to go all in and only eat salads. In fact, I like stir-fry dishes because you're getting your robust, substantial protein and marinades, which are only enhanced with plenty of veggies—like onions, snap peas, bok choy or whatever else you have on hand. Most grocery stores even sell kits of stir-fry veggies, already prepped for you. You really can't go wrong with whatever mix you decide on. As long as you have a good marinade, like a teriyaki or Thai peanut, you can make a variety of veggies (fresh or frozen!) taste amazing.

- ***Go crunchy and crispy.*** If these are your textures of choice, own it! Slice up some crisp cucumbers, daikon radish or peppers with a pinch of salt or dip, and eat like a chip. If you like food that's crispy, you'll love my crispy cabbage recipe in the back of this book and can have fun experimenting with brussels sprouts and turnip fries as well.

- ***Make soup or stew.*** If you have an immersion blender (or just a good blender), you can boil and blend up almost any veggie and broth into a soup or puree. It always tastes good.

PLATE IT!

AT THIS POINT, you've learned about the 2 Bunnies and the purpose of each food group. Now's the fun part when we put it all on a plate and see what you're going to be eating for all your meals. You'll still look at all your breakfasts, lunches and dinners as enjoyable. Plate It! makes them purposeful.

It's so simple. Nothing to weigh or measure. Just use the ratios below as a guide to each of your meals and you'll be full and satisfied, and energized and on track to meet your goals.

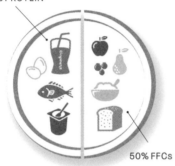

50% PROTEIN

50% FFCs

50% VEGGIES

25% PROTEIN

25% FFCs

Breakfast

- Water First! Aim for 16 fl. oz.** before your first bite
- In the morning you need 50% protein to help keep you full and 50% FFCs to give you lasting energy
- Veggies are extra credit; if you're hungrier in the mornings, they'll help make you full
- Accessorize as desired to make your meal delicious
- Find something quick and easy, that you love (like your favorite Shakeology recipe) and make it part of your consistent daily breakfast.

*Shakeology can be part of a healthy breakfast.

Lunch

- Water First! Aim for 16 fl. oz. before your first bite
- To keep you full and energized in the afternoon you need 50% veggies to make you full, 25% protein to help keep you full, and 25% FFCs to give you sustained energy
- Accessorize as desired to make your meal pop with flavor!

*Start with a smaller plate (7" to 9");
you can always go back for more if you're still hungry!*

TO RECAP, YOU'LL HAVE:

Veggies: Make us full and satisfied

Proteins: Keep us full and satisfied

Fiber-Filled Carbs: Give us sustained energy and are best for weight loss

Accessories: Get us eating more veggies and make our meals pop with flavor

Watch
The Video

Snack(tional)

- A snack is optional
- If you're going to have a snack, it should be between lunch and dinner
- Water First! Aim for 16 fl. oz. before your first bite
- Start with veggies
- If you need help to stay fuller longer, add a protein
- If you're still hungry and need more energy, add an FFC

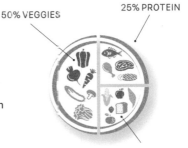

50% VEGGIES   25% PROTEIN

25% FFCs

Dinner

- Water First! Aim for 16 fl. oz. before your first bite
- Your plate should be 75% veggies to get full and 25% protein to help stay full
- Most people don't need additional energy at night, so there's no need to have an FFC at dinner
- Accessorize as desired to make your meal more comforting and delicious
- Remember once you've finished eating, it's "Dinner and Done" and time to move on with your night

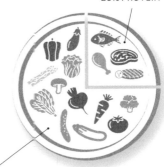

25% PROTEIN

75% VEGGIES

CHAPTER SUMMARY

■ *Make veggies your first bite. The only way to successfully stay slim long term is to learn to love them. They're easy to make. They improve your gut health. And you can accessorize them with delicious toppings.*

■ *Proteins keep you full and satisfied, and can help you lean down while also helping you build muscle.*

■ *Yes, you can eat carbs! FFCs—"fiber-filled carbs"—take longer than other carbs to break down, providing long-lasting energy.*

■ *Silly carbs cause your blood sugar to rise naturally, leading to a crash. Enjoy these responsibly.*

■ *Accessories make everything taste better. Add certain fats, sugars, spices, condiments and boosts to flavor your meals.*

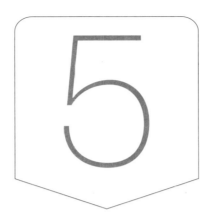

4-WEEK SLIM-DOWN PLAN

Melt Off the Weight in Just One Month
with This Step-by-Step Guide.

AM SO EXCITED for you to ease into the 2B Mindset and kick-start your weight loss with this exclusive 4-Week Slim-Down Plan. You'll utilize everything you learned in the previous chapters—Water First, Veggies Most, Use the Scale and Track—and to make it easy for you, I've even planned simple and delicious meals for each day.

Here are some tips to make the month go smoothly:

- Get in the 2B Mindset and tell yourself you're going to have fun this week. Enjoy new foods and lose some weight!

- Don't forget to drink water first before you eat.

- If you are ever still feeling hungry, be sure to reach for Water First and Veggies Most.

- If there's anything you feel like switching up—maybe you want to swap in a recipe from different weeks or want to try to incorporate Shakeology into your meal plan—do so now and adjust the grocery list accordingly.

- For best results, you will also want to record exactly what you're eating, how you're feeling and progressing in the 2B Mindset tracker. You can order the tracker and Shakeology, as well as get access to the videos and additional recipes, now at 2Bmindset.com, and start weaving them into your plan when they arrive in the next few days.

- Check your fridge, pantry and freezer for any items you may already have on the grocery list and cross them off.

Shake It Up This Month! *If you want a simple way to shake up any mealtime, check out our Shakeology recipes. Each one gives you suggestions on how to enjoy it as a breakfast, lunch or dinner! Chocolate is my favorite flavor. I even use it in recipes that sometimes call for other flavors like the birthday cake recipe on page 176 (it tastes like brownie batter!), but you can also get the sampler pack and mix and match to your liking.*

WEEK 1 OF 4

The stronger the start, the stronger you'll feel. Make this week great! If you want to eat some more, choose veggies as your first bite and remember: Veggies Most. Steamed, raw or baked veggies are great and can pair well with the Sweet and Savory Everything Sauce (see page 200) to be included as a snack or addition to dinner to help you achieve "dinner and done" and avoid late-night munchies.

Take time the day before you start the meal plan to do the following prep:

- *Wash and chop veggies.*

- *Make your Spiced Jumbo Burger patties and freeze two for next week.*

- *Spiralize zucchini "noodles" for your Spicy Peanut Sauce Over Zoodles.*

- *Cook spaghetti squash and use a fork to make "noodles" for your hash browns.*

- *If time permits, go ahead and make the Creamy Chicken Salad and/or the Bacon and Date Cabbage Salad.*

- *Make sure to store all this food in airtight containers in the fridge (or freezer for extras).*

Week 1 Meals

MINIMUM WATER GOAL

(Your weight in lbs. _____ ÷ 2 = _____ daily minimum goal in fluid ounces.)

	BREAKFAST	LUNCH	DINNER
Monday	Peanut Butter and Jelly Wonder Whip + an additional ¼ cup grapes	Creamy Chicken Salad + Bacon and Date Cabbage Salad + Whole-grain tortilla wrap * Tip 1	Baked Lemon Cod Packets + Tropical Mango Salad * Tip 4
Tuesday	Peanut Butter and Jelly Wonder Whip + an additional ¼ cup grapes	Spiced Jumbo Burger + Curried Cauliflower Risotto with Greens + ½ whole-grain hamburger bun * Tip 2	Lara's Baked Sesame Salmon + Bacon and Date Cabbage Salad * Tip 5
Wednesday	Peanut Butter and Jelly Wonder Whip + an additional ¼ cup grapes	Creamy Chicken Salad + Bacon and Date Cabbage Salad + Whole-grain tortilla wrap	Spiced Jumbo Burger + Curried Cauliflower Risotto with Greens
Thursday	Peanut Butter and Jelly Wonder Whip + an additional ¼ cup grapes	Spaghetti Squash Hash Browns + Tempeh Bacon + Prepared black bean soup * Tip 3	Lara's Baked Sesame Salmon + Kaitlin's Garlicky Carrots and Cauliflower Rice * Tip 6
Friday	Peanut Butter and Jelly Wonder Whip + an additional ¼ cup grapes	Spaghetti Squash Hash Browns + Tempeh Bacon + Prepared black bean soup	Eggplant Pizzas + lean ground turkey * Tip 7
Saturday	Tempeh Bacon + Whole-grain toast + ¼ Avocado	Spiced Jumbo Burger + Curried Cauliflower Risotto with Greens + ½ whole-grain hamburger bun	Garlic and Thyme Pressure Cooker Chicken + Spicy Peanut Sauce over Zoodles * Tip 8
Sunday	Tempeh Bacon + Whole-grain toast + ¼ Avocado	Garlic and Thyme Pressure Cooker Chicken + Kaitlin's Garlicky Carrots and Cauliflower Rice + cup hummus or ½ cup peas	Eggplant Pizzas + lean ground turkey

*TIPS

LUNCH

1. Creamy Chicken Salad
+ Bacon and Date Cabbage Salad
+ Whole-grain tortilla wrap

- Double the chicken salad recipe.

- Wrap both the chicken salad and cabbage salad into one tortilla or have the chicken salad with the tortilla and enjoy the salad on the side. If you want to add extra lettuce, tomato and/or onion to the tortilla, go ahead!

- Remember the tips for buying FFOs.

2. Spiced Jumbo Burger
+ Curried Cauliflower Risotto
with Greens + ½ whole-grain
hamburger bun

- Freeze four leftover burger patties to use next week. Enjoy two patties fresh today, two for dinner tomorrow and two for lunch on Saturday.

- Freeze leftover hamburger buns to use in week four.

- Triple the risotto recipe and serve with dinner tomorrow and lunch on Saturday.

3. Spaghetti Squash Hash Browns +
Tempeh Bacon + Prepared black bean
soup

- Cut the hash browns recipe in half

DINNER

4. Baked Lemon Cod Packets
+ Tropical Mango Salad

- Double the cod recipe and eat both servings for plenty of satisfying protein.

- Cut the mango salad recipe in half.

5. Lara's Baked Sesame Salmon
+ Bacon and Date Cabbage Salad

- Double the salmon recipe. Serve the other portion for dinner on Thursday.

- Plate two servings of cabbage salad.

6. Lara's Baked Sesame Salmon
+ Kaitlin's Garlicky Carrots and
Cauliflower Rice

- Double the cauliflower recipe and serve the other portion with lunch on Sunday.

7. Eggplant Pizzas + lean ground turkey

- Cut the pizza recipe in half to make 2 servings. Serve the second portion for dinner on Sunday.

- Cook 10 ounces of ground turkey in a separate skillet until no longer pink. Add to the sauce in step 5 of the eggplant recipe.

8. Garlic and Thyme Pressure
Cooker Chicken + Spicy Peanut Sauce
over Zoodles

- Use both servings of zoodles tonight!

- Shred the chicken and add to the zoodles.

GROCERY LIST–*WEEK 1*

PRODUCE

2 small apples

1 medium avocado

4 oz. baby mixed greens
(spinach, chard and kale)

1 bunch fresh basil leaves

4 oz. fresh bean sprouts

1 medium orange bell pepper

2 medium red bell peppers

1 medium yellow bell pepper

2 bags (14 oz. each) shredded
green cabbage (or coleslaw mix)

4 small carrots

5 bags (10 oz. each)
+ 1 (14-oz.) bag cauliflower rice

1 bunch celery

1 bunch fresh cilantro

1 medium eggplant

2 heads garlic

1 lb. red grapes

4 medium lemons

1 head lettuce

1 head romaine lettuce

1 medium lime

1 medium mango

1 bunch fresh mint

6 medium onions

1 medium red onion

1 bunch green onions

1 large orange

1 bunch fresh parsley

4 oz. fresh (or frozen) peas

4 medium shallots

1 small (2-lb.) spaghetti squash

4 medium zucchini

1 container fresh thyme

PROTEIN AND DAIRY

1 package center-cut bacon

1 oz. shredded Italian blend cheese

1 container spreadable cheese

8 oz. cooked or 11 oz. raw boneless,
skinless chicken breast

2 (4 oz. each) boneless, skinless
frozen chicken breasts

8 oz. raw cod fillet

8 oz. raw salmon fillet

1 (8-oz.) package tempeh

1 lb. 10 oz. raw 93% lean ground
turkey

1 (32-oz.) container + 1 (8-oz.)
container + 1 (4-oz.) container
plain reduced-fat (2%) Greek
yogurt

DRY AND PACKAGED FOODS

1 (16-oz.) container all-natural black bean soup

1 loaf whole-grain (or whole wheat) bread (Tip: Freeze loaf after using for weeks 2–4.)

1 (12-oz.) container low-sodium organic vegetable broth

2 oz. unsweetened shredded coconut

3 Medjool dates

1 jar all-natural fig preserves

1 whole-grain hamburger bun

1 oz. unsalted peanuts

1 (4-oz.) can all-natural tomato sauce, no salt or sugar added

2 whole-grain tortilla wraps

PANTRY

Ground cinnamon (optional)

Chili powder

Ground coriander

Ground cumin

Curry powder

Garlic powder

Ground ginger

Honey

Hot pepper sauce (like Sriracha™)

Dried Italian seasoning

Pure maple syrup

All-natural mayonnaise

Mustard

Olive oil

Sesame oil

Onion powder

Ground smoked paprika

Peanut butter powder

Ground black pepper

Crushed red pepper flakes (optional)

Sea salt (or Himalayan salt)

Sesame seeds (white or black)

Reduced-sodium soy sauce

Liquid stevia (optional)

Pure vanilla extract

Apple cider vinegar

Rice wine vinegar

BAKING SUPPLIES

Aluminum foil

Nonstick cooking spray

Parchment paper

WEEK 2 OF 4

Keep it up; this week is your chance to accelerate your goals! Take time the day before you start the meal plan to do the following prep:

- *Wash and chop veggies (Water First, Veggies Most if hungry).*

- *Cook quinoa (or buy it precooked). If you have extra, freeze it for next week.*

- *Remember to defrost your leftover Spiced Jumbo Burger patties from last week the night before to enjoy for dinner Wednesday and lunch on Friday.*

- *If time permits, go ahead and make the Citrus Marinated Tofu, Quick and Easy Citrus Slaw and/or Baked Zucchini Packets.*

- *Make sure to store all this food in airtight containers in the fridge (or freezer for extras).*

Week 2 Meals

MINIMUM WATER GOAL

(Your weight in lbs. _____ ÷ 2 = _____ daily minimum goal in fluid ounces.)

	BREAKFAST	LUNCH	DINNER
Monday	BEACHBAR Breakfast Bowl	Citrus Marinated Tofu + Quick and Easy Citrus Slaw + 1 small orange * Tip 1	Baked Lemon Cod Packets + Baked Zucchini Packets with Tomato and Herbs * Tip 6
Tuesday	BEACHBAR Breakfast Bowl	Baked Lemon Cod Packets + Baked Zucchini Packets with Tomato and Herbs + Quinoa	Citrus Marinated Tofu + Quick and Easy Citrus Slaw * Tip 7
Wednesday	BEACHBAR Breakfast Bowl	Garlic and Thyme Pressure Cooker Chicken + Spaghetti Squash Taco Boats + ½ cup black beans * Tip 2	Spiced Jumbo Burger + Eggplant Sandwich Thins * Tip 8
Thursday	BEACHBAR Breakfast Bowl	Citrus Marinated Tofu + Quick and Easy Citrus Slaw + 1 small orange	Garlic and Thyme Pressure Cooker Chicken + Spaghetti Squash Taco Boats * Tip 9
Friday	BEACHBAR Breakfast Bowl	Spiced Jumbo Burger + Eggplant Sandwich Thins + corn on the cob * Tip 3	Grilled chicken + Cheesy Tomato Noodle Soup * Tip 10
Saturday	Cheesy Egg White, Kale and Mushroom Pizza + 1 slice whole grain toast	Ground turkey + Spaghetti Squash Taco Boats + ½ cup black beans * Tip 4	Lara's Baked Sesame Salmon + Big salad * Tip 11
Sunday	Cheesy Egg White, Kale and Mushroom Pizza + 1 slice whole grain toast	Grilled chicken + Cheesy Tomato Noodle Soup + ½ cup black beans * Tip 5	Cheesy Cabbage Steak Turkey Sandwich

*TIPS

LUNCH

1. Citrus Marinated Tofu + Quick and Easy Citrus Slaw + 1 small orange

- Double the slaw recipe to make four servings.

2. Garlic and Thyme Pressure Cooker Chicken + Spaghetti Squash Taco Boats + ½ cup black beans

- Double the taco boat recipe to make four servings.
- See the tip for Saturday's lunch for a fun spin on the taco boats.

3. Spiced Jumbo Burger + Eggplant Sandwich Thins + corn on the cob

- Place each patty between two slices of eggplant sandwich thins to create two small sandwiches.

4. Ground turkey + Spaghetti Squash Taco Boats + ½ cup black beans

- Add the cooked ground turkey and black beans to one of the spaghetti squash taco boats before baking or scoop out the mixture from the squash skin and serve everything combined in a bowl.

5. Grilled chicken + Cheesy Tomato Noodle Soup + ½ cup black beans

- Add the black beans to the soup or serve on the side; your choice!

DINNER

6. Baked Lemon Cod Packets + Baked Zucchini Packets with Tomato and Herbs

- Triple the cod recipe and eat two servings for plenty of satisfying protein tonight and one serving for lunch tomorrow.

7. Citrus Marinated Tofu + Quick and Easy Citrus Slaw

- Serve yourself two portions of citrus slaw to be Veggies Most and keep you satisfied so you can be Dinner and Done!

8. Spiced Jumbo Burger + Eggplant Sandwich Thins

- Defrost your leftover patties from last week the night before to enjoy for dinner tonight and lunch on Friday.
- Cut the eggplant recipe in half to make only 4 servings (8 slices).
- Chop up the burger and divide evenly over two servings of the Eggplant Sandwich Thins and accessorize to your liking!

9. Garlic and Thyme Pressure Cooker Chicken + Spaghetti Squash Taco Boats

- Serve yourself two portions of the spaghetti squash taco boats.

10. Grilled chicken + Cheesy Tomato Noodle Soup

- Cut the soup recipe in half to make only two servings.

11. Lara's Baked Sesame Salmon + Big salad

- Use all of your leftover veggies to make a large salad and top with your favorite dressing or keep it simple with oil and vinegar or lemon juice, salt and pepper. Serve salmon on top or on the side.

GROCERY LIST—WEEK 2

PRODUCE

1 medium avocado

2 medium green bell peppers

3 medium red bell peppers

2 bags (14 oz. each) shredded green cabbage (or coleslaw mix)

1 medium red cabbage

2 small carrots

1 bunch celery

1 bunch fresh cilantro

1 lb. 4 oz. prepared low-sodium coleslaw

1 ear corn on the cob

1 medium eggplant

1 head garlic

1 (5-oz.) bag chopped kale

2 medium lemons

1 (5-oz.) bag lettuce

8 medium limes

2 containers (8 oz. each) mushrooms

1 (8-oz.) container sliced mushrooms

3 medium onions

1 medium red onion

2 small oranges

1 bunch fresh parsley

2 small (approx. 2 lb. each) spaghetti squash

2 medium zucchini squash

2 containers (16 oz. each) + 1 (8-oz.) container fresh strawberries or 2 bags frozen strawberries

1 container fresh thyme

2 medium tomatoes

2 small tomatoes

PROTEIN AND DAIRY

2 oz. finely shredded cheddar cheese

3 oz. shredded part-skim mozzarella cheese

12 oz. grilled or 1 lb. raw boneless, skinless chicken breast

2 (4 oz. each) boneless, skinless frozen chicken breasts

12 oz. raw cod fillet

8 large eggs or 1 cup egg whites

4 oz. raw salmon fillet

1 (14-oz.) package extra firm tofu

5 oz. raw 93% lean ground turkey

6 oz. nitrate- and nitrite-free deli turkey slices

1 (32-oz.) container plain reduced fat (2%) Greek yogurt

GROCERY LIST–*WEEK 2 cont'd*

DRY AND PACKAGED FOODS

5 BEACHBARS, any flavor

1 (15-oz.) can black beans

1 loaf whole-grain (or whole wheat) bread (see tip on week 1)

1 jar all-natural marinara sauce or use all-natural marinara sauce with basil (below)

1 jar all-natural marinara sauce with basil

2 oz. dry quinoa

2 packages (1 oz. each) low-sodium taco seasoning

2 bags (8 oz. each) tofu shirataki noodles

1 (16-oz.) box all-natural tomato soup

PANTRY

Ground coriander

Ground cumin

Garlic powder

Dried Italian seasoning

Olive oil

Sesame oil

Onion powder

Dried oregano

Ground paprika

Ground black pepper

Salad dressing (pick your favorite) or balsamic (or red wine) vinegar

Sea salt (or Himalayan salt)

Sesame seeds (white or black)

Reduced-sodium soy sauce

BAKING SUPPLIES

Aluminum foil

Nonstick cooking spray

Parchment paper

WEEK 3 OF 4

You're doing amazing. Remember, the more effort you put in, the more effortless it'll become. Take time the day before you start the meal plan to do the following prep:

- *Wash and chop veggies.*

- *If you loved the Bacon and Date Cabbage Salad, make it as part of your weekday breakfasts.*

- *Break out your slow cooker and whip up a large batch of Slow Cooker Veggies Most and Beef Chili. You'll be having half this week and the other half in week four, so store those other three servings properly in the freezer.*

- *If time permits, go ahead and make your Eggroll in a Bowl recipe. Be sure to double it so you can have it for lunch on Monday and dinner on Tuesday.*

- *Make sure to store all this food in airtight containers in the fridge (or freezer for extras).*

Week 3 Meals

MINIMUM WATER GOAL

(Your weight in lbs. _____ ÷ 2 = _____ daily minimum goal in fluid ounces.)

	BREAKFAST	**LUNCH**	**DINNER**
Monday	Bacon and Date Cabbage Salad + 2 eggs (any style) + whole-grain toast * Tip 1	Eggroll in a Bowl + Lara's Baked Sesame Salmon + Small baked sweet potato (or ½ a large one) * Tip 3	Slow Cooker Veggies Most and Beef Chili + Cauliflower Steaks with Red Pepper Sauce * Tip 7
Tuesday	Bacon and Date Cabbage Salad + 2 eggs (any style) + whole-grain toast	Slow Cooker Veggies Most and Beef Chili + Cauliflower Steaks with Red Pepper Sauce + ½ cup cooked corn * Tip 4	Eggroll in a Bowl + Lara's Baked Sesame Salmon
Wednesday	Bacon and Date Cabbage Salad + 2 eggs (any style) + whole-grain toast	Slow Cooker Veggies Most and Beef Chili + Cauliflower Steaks with Red Pepper Sauce + ½ cup cooked corn * Tip 5	Citrus Marinated Tofu + Quick and Easy Citrus Slaw * Tip 8
Thursday	Bacon and Date Cabbage Salad + 2 eggs (any style) + whole-grain toast	Tempeh Bacon, Lettuce, and Tomato Sandwich + whole-grain sandwich slim + Noah's Animal Style Cauliflower * Tip 6	Creamy Chicken Salad + Quick and Easy Citrus Slaw * Tip 9
Friday	Bacon and Date Cabbage Salad + 2 eggs (any style) + whole-grain toast	Tempeh Bacon, Lettuce, and Tomato Sandwich + whole-grain sandwich slim + Noah's Animal Style Cauliflower	Cheesy Cabbage Steak Turkey Sandwich * Tip 10
Saturday	Oatmeal + Tempeh Bacon * Tip 2	Cheesy Cabbage Steak Turkey Sandwich + Small baked sweet potato (or ½ a large one)	Creamy Chicken Salad + Quick and Easy Citrus Slaw
Sunday	Oatmeal + Tempeh Bacon	Creamy Chicken Salad + A serving of berries or fruit + Quick and Easy Citrus Slaw	Citrus Marinated Tofu + big bowl of salad * Tip 11

*TIPS

BREAKFAST

1. Bacon and Date Cabbage Salad + 2 eggs (any style) + whole-grain toast

- Make one and a half times the cabbage salad recipe for a total of 6 servings.

- Divide those six servings into five portions to eat for breakfast each weekday morning.

- Serve with your favorite type of eggs (scrambled, poached, sunny side up!) and a side of toast.

2. Oatmeal + Tempeh Bacon

- Top your oatmeal with cinnamon, nuts and/or seeds to keep it fun and exciting.

LUNCH

3. Eggroll in a Bowl + Lara's Baked Sesame Salmon + Small baked sweet potato (or ½ a large one)

- Double both recipes to make 2 servings each.

4. Slow Cooker Veggies Most and Beef Chili + Cauliflower Steaks with Red Pepper Sauce + ½ cup cooked corn

- Add cooked corn to your chili for your FFC.

5. Slow Cooker Veggies Most and Beef Chili + Cauliflower Steaks with Red Pepper Sauce + ½ cup cooked corn

- Add cooked corn to your chili for your FFC.

6. Tempeh Bacon, Lettuce, and Tomato Sandwich + whole-grain sandwich slim + Noah's Animal Style Cauliflower

- To make a TBLT, spread mustard on one half of a sandwich thin, then layer tempeh bacon, lettuce and tomato, and top with second sandwich thin half.

- Cut the cauliflower recipe in half to make only two servings.

DINNER

7. Slow Cooker Veggies Most and Beef Chili + Cauliflower Steaks with Red Pepper Sauce

- Make the whole chili recipe, but freeze 3 servings for next week.

- Serve up two cauliflower steaks with your chili tonight.

8. Citrus Marinated Tofu + Quick and Easy Citrus Slaw

- Make the full recipe of the tofu, but plate 1 ½ servings for dinner tonight and the other 1 ½ for Sunday's dinner.

- Double the citrus slaw recipe to make four servings.

9. Creamy Chicken Salad + Quick and Easy Citrus Slaw

- Triple the chicken salad recipe to make three servings.

- Peel the leaves off a romaine lettuce head and wrap up the chicken salad in it. Yum!

10. Cheesy Cabbage Steak Turkey Sandwich

- Make 2 servings to make lunch tomorrow quick 'n' easy.

11. Citrus Marinated Tofu + big bowl of salad

- Use all of your leftover veggies to make one big "everything but the kitchen sink salad." Top with citrus marinated tofu.

GROCERY LIST–*WEEK 3*

PRODUCE

3 small apples

1 small container fresh berries
(any variety)

4 medium green bell peppers

2 medium red bell peppers

5 bags (14 oz. each) shredded
green cabbage (or coleslaw mix)

2 medium red cabbages

3 medium carrots

2 large heads cauliflower

1 bunch celery

1 bunch fresh cilantro

2 bags (14 oz. each) coleslaw mix
(or shredded green cabbage)

1 lb. 4 oz. low-sodium prepared
coleslaw

8 oz. fresh (or frozen) corn

1 daikon radish

2 heads garlic

4 medium lemons

1 head + 1 (5-oz.) bag lettuce

6 medium limes

3 medium onions

1 small red onion

1 bunch green onions

2 medium shallots

1 container fresh thyme

2 medium tomatoes

2 small sweet potatoes (or 1 large)

PROTEIN AND DAIRY

1 package center-cut bacon

1 lb. 95% lean ground beef

4 oz. shredded cheddar cheese

1 oz. grated Parmesan cheese

12 oz. cooked or 1 lb. raw boneless,
skinless chicken breast

10 each or 1 dozen large eggs

8 oz. raw salmon fillet

1 (8-oz.) package tempeh

1 (14-oz.) package extra firm tofu

12 oz. nitrate- and nitrite-free deli
turkey slices

1 (8-oz.) container plain reduced-
fat (2%) Greek yogurt

DRY AND PACKAGED FOODS

2 cans (15 oz. each) kidney (or pinto) beans or a combination of both

1 (16-oz.) jar roasted red bell peppers

1 loaf whole-grain (or whole wheat) bread (see tip on week 1)

5 Medjool dates

1 jar all-natural fig preserves

2 oz. nuts, unsalted, any variety (optional)

1 container oatmeal

1 jar butter pickles

1 package whole-grain sandwich thins

1 (1-oz.) package low-sodium taco seasoning

1 (28-oz.) can diced tomatoes, no salt added

1 oz. walnuts, unsalted

PANTRY

Bay leaves

Ground cinnamon (optional)

Chili powder

Ground coriander

Ground cumin

Garlic powder

Ground ginger

All-natural ketchup

Pure maple syrup

All-natural mayonnaise

Mustard

Olive oil

Sesame oil

Onion powder

Dried oregano

Ground paprika

Ground smoked paprika

Ground black pepper

Ground cayenne pepper (optional)

Crushed red pepper flakes (optional)

Sea salt (or Himalayan salt)

Sesame seeds (white or black)

Reduced-sodium soy sauce

Apple cider vinegar

Rice wine vinegar

BAKING SUPPLIES

Aluminum foil

Nonstick cooking spray

Parchment paper

WEEK 4 OF 4

If you've stumbled at all, make it part of the dance. You can do this; have a great final week! Take time the day before you start the meal plan to do the following prep:

- *Wash and chop veggies.*

- *Remember to move your frozen Slow Cooker Veggies Most and Beef Chili into the fridge so it's thawed and ready to be heated on Monday night.*

- *Pre-cook your grilled chicken for Monday and Thursday's lunch.*

- *While the grill is hot, go ahead and make the Grilled Marinated Eggplant with Tahini Sauce.*

- *If you have more time, go ahead and make the Baked Zucchini Packets with Tomato and Herbs. Note that this recipe can also be made on an outdoor grill.*

- *Make sure to store all this food in airtight containers in the fridge (or freezer for extras).*

Week 4 Meals

MINIMUM WATER GOAL

(Your weight in lbs. _____ ÷ 2 = _____ daily minimum goal in fluid ounces.)

	BREAKFAST	LUNCH	DINNER
Monday	Peanut Butter and Jelly Wonder Whip + ½ small banana	Grilled chicken + Grilled Marinated Eggplant with Tahini Sauce + whole-grain pita bread * Tip 2	Slow Cooker Veggies Most and Beef Chili + Baked Zucchini Packets with Tomato and Herbs * Tip 8
Tuesday	Peanut Butter and Jelly Wonder Whip + ½ small banana	Slow Cooker Veggies Most and Beef Chili + ½ cup corn + Baked Zucchini Packets with Tomato and Herbs * Tip 3	Lara's Baked Sesame Salmon + Crispy Cabbage * Tip 9
Wednesday	Peanut Butter and Jelly Wonder Whip + ½ small banana	Slow Cooker Veggies Most and Beef Chili + ½ cup corn + Baked Zucchini Packets with Tomato and Herbs	Lara's Baked Sesame Salmon + Crispy Cabbage
Thursday	Peanut Butter and Jelly Wonder Whip + ½ small banana	Grilled chicken + Grilled Marinated Eggplant with Tahini Sauce + whole-grain pita bread * Tip 4	Veggie Burger Patty + Curried Cauliflower Risotto with Greens * Tip 10
Friday	Peanut Butter and Jelly Wonder Whip + ½ small banana	Spaghetti Squash Carbonara + Tempeh Bacon * Tip 5	Baked Lemon Cod Packets + Cheesy Tomato Noodle Soup * Tip 11
Saturday	Spaghetti Squash Carbonara + Tempeh Bacon + whole-grain toast + ¼ avocado * Tip 1	Veggie Burger Patty + Black beans + Curried Cauliflower Risotto with Greens * Tip 6	Garlic and Thyme Pressure Cooker Chicken + Spicy Peanut Sauce over Zoodles * Tip 12
Sunday	Spaghetti Squash Carbonara + 2 sunny-side up eggs + whole-grain toast	Baked Lemon Cod Packets + Cheesy Tomato Noodle Soup + black beans * Tip 7	Garlic and Thyme Pressure Cooker Chicken + Spicy Peanut Sauce over Zoodles

*TIPS

BREAKFAST

1. Spaghetti Squash Carbonara + Tempeh Bacon + whole-grain toast + ¼ avocado

- Crumble tempeh bacon on top of carbonara. Spread avocado on toast.

LUNCH

2. Grilled chicken + Grilled Marinated Eggplant with Tahini Sauce + whole-grain pita bread

- Remember your tips for buying FFCs.

3. Slow Cooker Veggies Most and Beef Chili + ½ cup corn + Baked Zucchini Packets with Tomato and Herbs

- Add cooked corn to your chili for your FFC.

4. Grilled chicken + Grilled Marinated Eggplant with Tahini Sauce + whole-grain pita bread

- Remember your tips for buying FFCs.

5. Spaghetti Squash Carbonara + Tempeh Bacon

- Plate two servings of spaghetti squash for lunch and reserve the other two for your weekend breakfasts.
- Cut the tempeh bacon recipe in half to make only two servings.

6. Veggie Burger Patty + Black beans + Curried Cauliflower Risotto with Greens

- Choose a veggie burger with at least 10 g protein

7. Baked Lemon Cod Packets + Cheesy Tomato Noodle Soup + black beans

- Add ½ cup cooked black beans to your soup as your FFC.

DINNER

8. Slow Cooker Veggies Most and Beef Chili + Baked Zucchini Packets with Tomato and Herbs

- Remember to move your frozen chili into the fridge the night before so it's thawed and ready to be heated.
- Double the zucchini recipe to make four servings. Plate two for dinner tonight.

9. Lara's Baked Sesame Salmon + Crispy Cabbage

- Double both recipes to make dinner tomorrow super simple.

10. Veggie Burger Patty + Curried Cauliflower Risotto with Greens

- Choose a veggie burger with at least 10 g protein.
- Double the risotto recipe to make two servings.
- Use the outer leaves to wrap the burger in a lettuce bun and add additional sliced tomato and onion to your liking

11. Baked Lemon Cod Packets + Cheesy Tomato Noodle Soup

- Make 3 servings of cod and plate two for dinner tonight and one for lunch on Sunday.
- Cut the soup recipe in half to make only two servings.

12. Garlic and Thyme Pressure Cooker Chicken + Spicy Peanut Sauce over Zoodles

- Double the zoodles recipe to make four servings. Plate two servings tonight and two for tomorrow's dinner.
- Shred chicken and add to zoodles.

GROCERY LIST–*WEEK 4*

PRODUCE

1 medium avocado

4 oz. baby mixed greens
(spinach, chard and kale)

3 small bananas

8 oz. fresh bean sprouts

2 medium red bell peppers

1 small carrot

2 bags (10-oz. each) cauliflower rice

1 bunch celery

1 bunch fresh cilantro

2 bags (12 oz. each) coleslaw mix
(or shredded green cabbage)

8 oz. fresh (or frozen) corn

1 medium globe eggplant

2 heads garlic

8 oz. red grapes

5 medium lemons

2 medium limes

4 medium onions

1 bunch green onions

1 bunch fresh parsley

1 small (approx. 2-lb.)
spaghetti squash

12 medium zucchini

1 container fresh thyme

4 medium tomatoes

PROTEIN AND DAIRY

2 oz. shredded part-skim
mozzarella cheese

1 oz. grated Parmesan cheese

1 container spreadable cheese

8 oz. cooked or 12 oz. raw boneless,
skinless chicken breast

2 (4 oz. each) boneless, skinless
frozen chicken breasts

12 oz. raw cod fillet

5 each or 1 dozen large eggs

8 oz. raw salmon fillet

1 (8-oz.) package tempeh

1 package veggie patties
(at least 10 grams of protein each)

1 (32-oz.) container + 1 (8-oz.)
container plain reduced-fat (2%)
Greek yogurt

GROCERY LIST–**WEEK 4 cont'd**

DRY AND PACKAGED FOODS

1 (15-oz.) can black beans

1 loaf whole-grain (or whole wheat) bread (see tip on week 1)

1 (12-oz.) container low-sodium vegetable broth

1 jar all-natural marinara sauce with basil

1 oz. unsalted peanuts

1 package whole-grain pita bread

1 jar tahini paste

1 (16-oz.) box all-natural tomato soup

2 bags (8 oz. each) tofu shirataki noodles

PANTRY

Ground cinnamon (optional)

Curry powder

Everything bagel seasoning blend

Garlic powder

Ground ginger

Honey

Hot pepper sauce (like Sriracha™)

Dried Italian seasoning

Pure maple syrup

Olive oil

Sesame oil

Onion powder

Ground smoked paprika

Peanut butter powder

Ground black pepper

Crushed red pepper flakes (optional)

Sea salt (or Himalayan salt)

Sesame seeds (white or black)

Reduced-sodium soy sauce

Liquid stevia (optional)

Pure vanilla extract

Rice wine vinegar

BAKING SUPPLIES

Aluminum foil

Nonstick cooking spray

Parchment paper

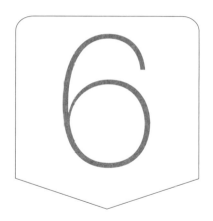

2B MINDSET RECIPES

50 Delicious Breakfasts,
Lunches, Dinners and More—
From C (Cabbage) to Z (Zucchini).

CABBAGE

BACON & DATE
CABBAGE SALAD

(Makes 4 servings, approx. 2 cups each)

TOTAL TIME: **15 MINUTES** / PREP TIME: **12 MINUTES** / COOKING TIME: **3 MINUTES**

Nonstick cooking spray

3 slices center-cut bacon (nitrate- and nitrite-free)

3 Tbsp. olive oil

1 medium shallot, thinly sliced

2 Tbsp. apple cider vinegar

1 Tbsp. all-natural fig preserves

1 Tbsp. fresh thyme leaves

2 (14-oz.) bags shredded cabbage (or coleslaw mix)

Sea salt (or Himalayan salt) and ground black pepper (to taste; optional)

3 Medjool dates, pitted and chopped

1. Heat oven to 400° F.

2. Line a small baking sheet with parchment paper; lightly coat it with cooking spray.

3. Arrange the bacon on the sheet in one layer. Bake for 15 to 20 minutes until crisp (or according to package directions); set aside.

4. While the bacon cooks, heat the oil in medium nonstick skillet over medium heat.

5. Add the shallot; cook, stirring frequently, 2 to 3 minutes, or until translucent. Remove from heat.

6. Add the vinegar, preserves and thyme; stir to make dressing. Set aside.

7. Place the cabbage in a large heatproof bowl; pour the warm dressing over cabbage. Mix the salad thoroughly; season with salt and pepper, if desired.

8. Garnish with the bacon and dates. Divide evenly among eight serving plates.

Tips

■ To make this a satisfying breakfast (with plenty of extra credit) top the salad with 2 eggs and pair with a toasted whole-grain English muffin.

■ To make this a yummy lunch option, pair it with a serving of Creamy Chicken Salad (see page 168) and a whole-grain toasted English muffin.

■ To make this a satisfying dinner, omit the English muffin from the lunch option and have one to two servings of the salad mixture to ensure you can be dinner and done!

■ Try this recipe with other fruit preserves (apricot, apple, blackcurrant, etc.).

CABBAGE

CABBAGE STEAKS
with Creamy Ranch Dressing
(Makes 5 servings, approx. 2 cabbage moons
and ¼ cup dressing each)

TOTAL TIME: **1 HOUR 10 MINUTES** / PREP TIME: **10 MINUTES** / COOKING TIME: **1 HOUR**

Parchment paper

Nonstick cooking spray

1   large red (or green) cabbage, cut in half lengthwise, sliced into ½-inch-thick moons (approx. 10 pieces)

½ tsp. garlic powder

½ tsp. onion powder

Sea salt (or Himalayan salt) and ground black pepper (to taste; optional)

1   cup reduced fat (2%) plain Greek yogurt

1   Tbsp. red wine vinegar

2   Tbsp. water

2   tsp. reduced sodium ranch seasoning mix

2   Tbsp. finely chopped red bell pepper

1. Preheat oven to 350°F.

2. Line a baking sheet with parchment paper and lightly coat with cooking spray.

3. Arrange the cabbage moons in a single layer on the baking sheet.

4. Sprinkle the cabbage with the garlic powder and onion powder. Season with salt and pepper, if desired.

5. Bake for 1 hour, or until the cabbage is tender; set aside.

6. To make the dressing, combine yogurt, vinegar, water, ranch seasoning and bell pepper in a medium bowl; whisk to blend.

7. Serve 2 pieces cabbage on a plate and drizzle with ¼ cup dressing; repeat for each serving. Store the remaining cabbage and dressing refrigerated in separate, airtight containers for up to four days.

Tips

■ You can substitute 2 medium cabbages for 1 large cabbage.

■ To make this recipe vegan, substitute unsweetened, plain coconut milk yogurt for Greek yogurt.

■ You can swap out ranch seasoning mix for reduced sodium onion soup mix and add parsley.

■ To make this a dinner, replace the bean-based soup with a veggie-based broth soup.

■ To make this a lunch, pair with a serving of Creamy Chicken Salad (see page 168) and a bean-based soup.

CABBAGE

CRISPY CABBAGE
(Makes 1 serving)

TOTAL TIME: **18 MINUTES** / PREP TIME: **3 MINUTES** / COOKING TIME: **15 MINUTES**

Parchment paper

Nonstick cooking spray

1   (14-oz.) bag coleslaw
    mix (or shredded
    cabbage) (approx.
    6 cups)

1   tsp. olive oil

2   Tbsp. everything bagel
    seasoning blend

Sea salt (or Himalayan
    salt) and ground
    black pepper (to taste;
    optional)

1. Preheat oven to 425° F.

2. Line two large baking sheets with
   parchment paper and lightly coat them
   with cooking spray.

3. Mix the coleslaw (or shredded cabbage,
   if using), olive oil and everything bagel
   seasoning blend in a medium bowl.

4. Evenly divide the cabbage mixture
   between the baking sheets, spreading in
   a thin layer to the edge of each sheet.

5. Bake 15 minutes, stirring once and rotating
   the baking sheets halfway through, until
   the cabbage is dry with crispy, brown edges.

6. Season with salt and pepper, to taste. Serve
   immediately.

Tips

- Everything bagel seasoning blend is a dry seasoning that may contain sesame seeds, poppy seeds,
  garlic, onion and possibly
  other seeds and spices.

- To make this a lunch, pair
  with one small roasted
  sweet potato and a serving
  of Lara's Baked Sesame
  Salmon (see page 170).

- To make this a dinner,
  omit the sweet potatoes
  from the lunch option.

- Using two baking sheets
  will keep the cabbage
  from steaming and allow
  it to crisp.

- Coleslaw mix contains
  vegetables only. If using
  a "kit," omit the provided
  dressing.

EGGROLL IN A BOWL
(Makes 1 serving)

TOTAL TIME: **11 MINUTES** / PREP TIME: **6 MINUTES** / COOKING TIME: **5 MINUTES**

Nonstick cooking spray

2 green onions, thinly sliced

¼ cup finely chopped red bell pepper

2 cloves garlic, finely chopped

¼ tsp. crushed red pepper flakes (optional)

1 (14-oz.) bag coleslaw mix (or shredded green cabbage)

¼ tsp. ground ginger

½ cup daikon radish, peeled, grated

1 tsp. rice wine vinegar

1 tsp. reduced-sodium soy sauce

½ tsp. sesame oil

1. Heat a large nonstick pan over high heat; lightly coat it with cooking spray.

2. Add the green onion, bell pepper, garlic and red pepper flakes; cook, stirring frequently, for 1 minute.

3. Add the coleslaw (or cabbage) and ginger; cook, stirring frequently, for 3 to 5 minutes, until the cabbage is tender.

4. Add the daikon, vinegar and soy sauce; cook 1 minute, stirring frequently.

5. Remove from heat and add the oil; stir. Serve immediately

Tips

■ Daikon is type of radish that looks like a very large white carrot. It can be found in the produce section of most grocery stores.

■ To make this a lunch, add ½ cup corn to step 3 above and pair with a serving of Lara's Baked Sesame Salmon recipe (see page 170).

■ Coleslaw mix contains vegetables only. If using a "kit" omit the provided dressing.

■ To make it a dinner, omit the corn from the suggested lunch option.

CABBAGE

QUICK & EASY CITRUS SLAW
(Makes 2 servings, approx. 2 cups each)

TOTAL TIME: **2 HOURS 6 MINUTES** / PREP TIME: **6 MINUTES** / COOKING TIME: **NONE**

10 oz. conventionally prepared deli-style coleslaw

1 (14-oz.) bag shredded cabbage (or coleslaw mix)

1 cup chopped red (or green) bell pepper

¼ cup chopped red onion

2 Tbsp. chopped fresh cilantro

1 Tbsp. finely chopped lime peel (lime zest)

2 Tbsp. fresh lime juice

Sea salt (or Himalayan salt) and ground black pepper (to taste; optional)

1. Place the coleslaw, cabbage (or coleslaw mix), bell pepper, onion, lime peel and juice in a gallon-size, resealable plastic bag; shake it well to combine.

2. Place the coleslaw mixture in refrigerator for 2 to 24 hours for flavors to meld.

3. Divide the mixture between two plates and serve, or store refrigerated in an airtight container for up to four days.

Tips

■ To make this a lunch pair with a serving of Citrus Marinated Tofu (see page 167) and one small orange for a refreshing summer meal.

■ If the prepared coleslaw is drenched in dressing, place it in a strainer to remove the excess before using. You can replace store-bought coleslaw with an additional bag of shredded cabbage and 3 Tbsp. coleslaw dressing diluted with 1–2 Tbsp. water.

■ To make this a dinner, omit the orange from the lunch suggestion and have one to two servings of the slaw to make sure you are full and satisfied.

CAULIFLOWER STEAKS
with Red Pepper Sauce
(Makes 4 servings, approx. 1 steak and ¼ cup sauce each)

TOTAL TIME: **1 HOUR 15 MINUTES** / PREP TIME: **15 MINUTES** / COOKING TIME: **1 HOUR**

Parchment paper

Nonstick cooking spray

1   large head cauliflower, leaves and stem removed, sliced lengthwise into 1-inch slices (approx. 4 steaks)

½   tsp. garlic powder

½   tsp. onion powder

Sea salt (or Himalayan salt) and ground black pepper (to taste; optional)

1   (16-oz.) jar roasted red peppers (packed in water), drained

1   clove garlic

1   Tbsp. grated Parmesan cheese

1   Tbsp. chopped walnuts, unsalted

1   Tbsp. red wine vinegar

1   tsp. ground smoked paprika

2   Tbsp. water (optional; if desired)

1. Preheat oven to 350°F.

2. Line the baking sheet with parchment paper; lightly coat it with cooking spray.

3. Arrange the cauliflower on the baking sheet in a single layer.

4. Sprinkle the cauliflower with garlic powder and onion powder; season with salt and black pepper, if desired.

5. Bake for 1 hour, or until the cauliflower is tender.

6. While the cauliflower bakes, place the red peppers, garlic, cheese, walnuts, vinegar and paprika in a food processor and pulse until smooth, about 1 minute; add 1 to 2 Tbsp. water, if needed, to thin sauce; set aside.

7. Divide the cauliflower evenly among four plates; top them evenly with the sauce, about ¼ cup each.

8. Serve immediately, or store refrigerated in an airtight container for up to four days.

Tips

■ You can substitute 2 small cauliflower for 1 large.

■ To make this a delicious lunch, pair two servings with 1 cup of the Slow Cooker Veggies Most and Beef Chili (see page 172) and add ½ cup cooked corn to the chili.

■ When slicing the cauliflower steaks, cut straight down through the whole head, being careful to not break off any florets, keeping each steak intact.

■ To make this a breakfast, chop the cauliflower steak and wrap it in a whole-grain tortilla with two scrambled eggs. Top with the red pepper sauce.

■ To enjoy as a dinner, remove the corn from the lunch option and have two to three servings of the cauliflower to make sure your plate is Veggies Most!

CAULIFLOWER

CURRIED CAULIFLOWER
RISOTTO with Greens

(Makes 1 serving)

TOTAL TIME: **17 MINUTES** / PREP TIME: **6 MINUTES** / COOKING TIME: **9 MINUTES**

1 tsp. olive oil

1 cup chopped onion (approx. 1 medium)

½ tsp. curry powder

2 cloves garlic, finely chopped

1 (10-oz.) bag cauliflower rice

½ cup low-sodium organic vegetable broth

1 cup baby mixed greens, chopped (spinach, chard and kale), packed

1 (¾-oz.) wedge spreadable cheese, broken into small pieces

Sea salt (or Himalayan salt) and ground black pepper (to taste; optional)

1. Heat the oil in medium nonstick skillet over medium-high heat.

2. Add the onion and curry powder; cook, stirring frequently, for 2 to 3 minutes, or until the onion softens.

3. Add the garlic; cook, stirring frequently, for 30 seconds.

4. Add the cauliflower and broth; bring to a simmer. Cook, stirring frequently, for 4 minutes.

5. Add the greens; cook, stirring frequently, for 2 minutes, or until the greens wilt and the cauliflower is tender.

6. Remove from heat; stir in the cheese and enjoy, or store refrigerated in an airtight container for up to four days.

Tips

■ If curry isn't your favorite flavor, replace it with an Italian seasoning blend or herbs de Provence.

■ To make this a lunch, pair with a Spiced Jumbo Burger (see page 173) placed on top of ½ of a whole-grain bun.

■ To make this a savory breakfast, add ½ cup cooked peas and top it with two over-easy eggs.

■ To make this a dinner, omit the bun from the lunch option.

CAULIFLOWER

KAITLIN'S GARLICKY CARROTS & CAULIFLOWER RICE

(Makes 1 serving)

TOTAL TIME: **9 MINUTES** / PREP TIME: **3 MINUTES** / COOKING TIME: **6 MINUTES**

Nonstick cooking spray

3 cloves garlic, finely chopped

1 (10-oz.) bag cauliflower rice

1 cup shredded carrots

¼ tsp. onion powder

1 tsp. chopped fresh parsley

Sea salt (or Himalayan salt) and ground black pepper (to taste; optional)

1. Heat a large nonstick skillet, lightly coated with cooking spray over high heat.

2. Add the garlic, cauliflower, carrots and onion powder; cook, stirring frequently, for 3 to 5 minutes, or until the vegetables are tender.

3. Add the parsley, and season with salt and pepper, if desired; cook, stirring frequently, for 1 minute.

4. Serve immediately, or store refrigerated in an airtight container for up to four days.

Tips

■ If you're using frozen cauliflower rice, add it to the skillet after step 1 to defrost for 4 to 5 minutes. Drain the excess liquid, and proceed with step 2.

■ You can make your own cauliflower rice by grating it with a box grater, or by pulsing in a food processor. Spread the raw, grated cauliflower on a baking sheet and freeze; transfer it to a resealable plastic freezer bag for storage.

■ To make this a lunch, add ½ cup peas to step 2 above and pair with a serving of the Garlic and Thyme Pressure Cooker Chicken (see page 169)

■ To make this a dinner, omit the peas from the lunch option.

GREEK STYLE ROASTED CAULIFLOWER
(Makes 4 servings, approx. 1 cup each)

TOTAL TIME: **45 MINUTES + 2 HOURS TO MARINATE**
PREP TIME: **15 MINUTES** / COOKING TIME: **30 MINUTES**

1   large head cauliflower, chopped into florets (approx. 6 cups)

½   cup kalamata olives, pitted, sliced in half

2   Tbsp. finely chopped lemon peel (lemon zest), divided

4   Tbsp. fresh lemon juice, divided

5   fresh oregano sprigs

4   cloves garlic, finely chopped

1   Tbsp. olive oil

Sea salt (or Himalayan salt) and ground black pepper (to taste; optional)

Parchment paper

¼   cup feta cheese, crumbled

1   tsp. fresh oregano leaves, finely chopped

1. Mix the cauliflower, olives, 1 Tbsp. lemon peel, 2 Tbsp. lemon juice, the oregano sprigs, garlic and olive oil in a glass mixing bowl; season with salt and pepper to taste, if desired.

2. Cover the mixture with plastic wrap and marinate in refrigerator for 1 to 2 hours (optional).

3. Preheat oven to 400° F.

4. Line a baking sheet with parchment paper; arrange the cauliflower mixture in a single layer on the sheet.

5. Bake for 30 minutes, or until the cauliflower is tender and starts to brown.

6. Mix the feta cheese, the remaining 1 Tbsp. lemon peel and the remaining 2 Tbsp. lemon juice in a small bowl; set aside.

7. Remove the oregano sprigs from the cauliflower mixture. Transfer to a serving dish.

8. Top with the feta cheese mixture and chopped oregano leaves. Serve immediately, or store refrigerated in an airtight container for up to four days.

Tips

- The white flesh inside a lemon peel is bitter. Remove only the peel, and avoid the pith, for the best flavor.

- To make this a satisfying lunch, pair two servings with a serving of Baked Lemon Cod Packets (see page 165) and add ½ cup cooked chickpeas to the cauliflower mixture.

- To make this a delicious dinner, omit the chickpeas from the lunch suggestion.

> CAULIFLOWER

NOAH'S ANIMAL STYLE CAULIFLOWER

(Makes 4 servings, approx. 1 cup each)

TOTAL TIME: **50 MINUTES** / PREP TIME: **15 MINUTES** / COOKING TIME: **35 MINUTES**

Parchment paper

Nonstick cooking spray

1 large head cauliflower, separated into florets (approx. 6 cups)

1 Tbsp.– 1 tsp. low-sodium taco seasoning, divided

2 Tbsp. reduced-fat (2%) plain Greek yogurt

2 Tbsp. all-natural mayonnaise

1 Tbsp. all-natural ketchup

2 Tbsp. finely chopped red bell pepper

2 Tbsp. finely chopped onion

1 Tbsp. chopped butter pickles

1 Tbsp. water

½ tsp. apple cider vinegar

1 pinch ground cayenne pepper (optional)

¾ cup shredded cheddar cheese, divided

1. Preheat oven to 400° F.

2. Line a baking sheet with the parchment paper; lightly coat it with cooking spray.

3. Place the cauliflower in a large bowl; coat it with cooking spray. Add 1 Tbsp. taco seasoning; mix well.

4. Arrange the cauliflower in a single layer on the prepared baking sheet; bake 25 minutes, until it is golden brown and soft.

5. While the cauliflower cooks, place the yogurt, mayonnaise, bell pepper, onion, pickle, vinegar and cayenne pepper (if desired), in a medium bowl; whisk to combine. Set aside.

6. Combine ½ cup of the cheese and the remaining 1 tsp. taco seasoning in a small bowl. Set aside.

7. Sprinkle the cheese mixture onto the cauliflower. Loosely cover it with foil; bake 8 to 10 minutes more, until cheese melts.

8. Sprinkle the remaining ¼ cup cheese over the cauliflower; set aside 1 minute until the cheese melts.

9. Spoon the dressing over the cauliflower and cheese. Divide evenly between 4 serving plates; serve immediately.

Tips

■ To make this extra special, top with sautéed onions.

■ To enjoy as an indulgent dinner, skip the beans from the lunch option.

■ Make this recipe your own by substituting your favorite homemade yogurt-based creamy dressing and a complementary cheese (e.g., ranch and pepper jack).

■ To make this a yummy lunch, top two servings with a serving of Tempeh Bacon (see page 174) and ½ cup cooked black beans.

EGGPLANT

EGGPLANT PIZZAS
(Makes 4 servings, approx. 5 rounds each)

TOTAL TIME: **30 MINUTES** / PREP TIME: **10 MINUTES** / COOKING TIME: **20 MINUTES**

Parchment paper

Nonstick cooking spray

1   medium eggplant, sliced into ¼-inch-thick rounds

Sea salt (or Himalayan salt) and ground black pepper (to taste; optional)

1   (8-oz.) can all-natural tomato sauce

1   tsp. dried Italian seasoning

½   tsp. garlic powder

½   tsp. onion powder

1   dash crushed red pepper flakes (optional)

¼   cup fresh basil leaves, thinly sliced

½   cup shredded Italian cheese blend

1. Preheat oven to 375° F.

2. Line two baking sheet with the parchment paper; lightly coat with cooking spray.

3. Arrange the eggplant slices on the sheets in a single layer; season with salt and pepper, if desired.

4. Bake the eggplant for 10 minutes; use a spatula to flip. Bake for an additional 3 to 5 minutes; watch closely to prevent burning; set aside. Leave the oven on.

5. Place a small saucepan over medium heat; add the tomato sauce, Italian seasoning, garlic powder, onion powder and red pepper flakes (if using); bring to a gentle boil, stirring constantly, about 3 minutes.

6. Spoon the sauce evenly over the eggplant slices; top them evenly with basil and cheese.

7. Bake for 2 minutes, until the cheese melts.

Tips

■ To thinly slice fresh basil, stack the large leaves, then roll up the leaf from tip to stem and slice. You will end up with long, curly slices.

■ To make this a satisfying lunch, pair one serving with a serving of the Garlic and Thyme Pressure Cooker Chicken recipe (see page 169) and a side of fruit.

■ To make this a filling dinner, skip the fruit from the lunch suggestion and have two servings of eggplant, so you are full and satisfied and can be dinner and done!

EGGPLANT

EGGPLANT ROLLATINI
(Makes 5 servings, approx. 3 pieces each)

TOTAL TIME: **1 HOUR 3 MINUTES** / PREP TIME: **25 MINUTES** / COOKING TIME: **48 MINUTES**

Parchment paper

Nonstick cooking spray

2 medium eggplants, sliced lengthwise into fifteen ¼-inch slices

½ tsp. sea salt (or Himalayan salt), divided

2 cups all-natural tomato sauce

1½ tsp. dried Italian seasoning

½ tsp. onion powder

½ tsp. garlic powder

tsp. crushed red pepper flakes (optional)

Ground black pepper (to taste; optional)

1 (10-oz.) package frozen chopped spinach, thawed, squeezed dry

½ cup reduced-fat (2%) cottage cheese

½ cup shredded Italian cheese blend

Tips

- When squeezing the spinach, you will have removed enough water when the spinach fits in a ½-cup measure.

- If you over-reduce the tomato sauce, just add water to make 1½ cups.

1. Preheat oven to 400°F.

2. Line three baking sheets with the parchment paper (or work in batches, if needed); lightly coat with cooking spray.

3. Arrange the eggplant slices on the sheets in a single layer; sprinkle with ¼ tsp. salt. Bake for 10 minutes, until softened. Remove the eggplant from the sheet pans; set aside.

4. Heat a medium nonstick skillet over medium-high heat; add the tomato sauce, Italian seasoning, onion powder, garlic powder and red pepper flakes (if using). Cook, stirring constantly, for 5 minutes.

5. Reduce the heat to low and gently boil, stirring occasionally, until the sauce is reduced to about 1½ cups, about 10 minutes. Season with remaining ¼ tsp. salt, and pepper, if desired. Set aside.

6. Combine the spinach and cottage cheese in a medium bowl; mix well.

7. When the eggplant is cool enough to handle, spoon approximately 1 Tbsp. of the spinach mixture onto the wide end of an eggplant slice; roll up the eggplant from the wide end to the narrow end. Repeat until all the remaining spinach mixture and eggplant are used.

8. Evenly spread half of the tomato sauce mixture in 9 x 14-inch baking dish. Arrange the eggplant rolls, seam-side down, in a baking dish, leaving space between each roll; spoon the remaining tomato sauce mixture over each roll. Bake for 20 to 25 minutes, until the sauce bubbles.

9. Top the rolls evenly with the cheese. Bake for 2 to 3 minutes more, until the cheese melts.

10. Divide the rolls evenly between five plates, about 3 rolls each, or store refrigerated in an airtight container up to four days.

EGGPLANT

EGGPLANT SANDWICH THINS
(Makes 8 servings, approx. 2 slices each)

TOTAL TIME: **35 MINUTES** / PREP TIME: **5 MINUTES** / COOKING TIME: **30 MINUTES**

Parchment paper

Nonstick cooking spray

1 medium eggplant, sliced into ¼-inch-thick rounds (approx. 16 rounds)

Sea salt (or Himalayan salt) and ground black pepper (to taste; optional)

1. Preheat oven to 375° F.

2. Line 1 or 2 large baking sheets with the parchment paper and lightly coat with cooking spray.

3. Arrange the eggplant on the baking sheets in a single layer; leave space between the slices and do not overlap.

4. Season with salt and pepper.

5. Bake 25 to 30 minutes, flipping after 15 minutes, until the eggplant is mostly dry. Immediately transfer to a cooling rack, and allow to cool fully before storing.

Tips

■ Use the thins to make sandwiches with ¼ mashed avocado and sea salt, hummus and crumbled feta, or cream cheese made with Greek yogurt and finely chopped chives, or your favorite sandwich ingredients.

■ Store fully cooled slices, refrigerated in an airtight container, separated by squares of parchment paper, for up to three days.

■ To make this a lunch, place a Spiced Jumbo Burger (see page 173) between two sandwich thins and pair with a side of Crispy Cabbage (see page 152) and corn on the cob.

■ Reheat the slices in a toaster oven, if desired. Do not use a vertical bread toaster.

■ To make this a yummy dinner, omit the corn on the cob from the lunch recommendation and have two servings of eggplant so your plate is Veggies Most.

EGGPLANT

GRILLED MARINATED EGGPLANT with Tahini Sauce

(Makes 2 servings, approx. 1½ cup each)

TOTAL TIME: **14 MINUTES + 1 HOUR TO MARINATE** /
PREP TIME: **8 MINUTES** / COOKING TIME: **6 MINUTES**

1 medium eggplant, halved lengthwise, sliced ⅓-inch thick

Sea salt (or Himalayan salt) and ground black pepper (to taste; optional)

¼ cup + 2 Tbsp. fresh lemon juice, divided

2 cloves garlic, finely chopped, divided

1 Tbsp. tahini paste

1 tsp. honey

2 Tbsp. hot water

¼ cup chopped fresh parsley

1. Preheat a grill or grill pan over high heat.

2. Season the eggplant slices with salt and pepper side, until grill marks form; remove from heat and transfer the slices to a shallow baking dish.

3. Mix ¼ cup lemon juice with 1 clove garlic; pour the lemon mixture over the eggplant. Cover with a tightly fitted lid or plastic wrap, so that steam builds up and the eggplant softens. Place in refrigerator for at least 1 hour, or overnight.

4. Whisk the remaining 2 Tbsp. lemon juice, the remaining 1 clove garlic, the tahini, honey, water, and salt and pepper, if desired, in a small bowl; set aside.

5. Divide the eggplant evenly between two plates; drizzle with the tahini mixture and garnish with the parsley. Serve immediately, or store refrigerated in an airtight container for up to four days.

Tips

- To get good grill marks on the eggplant, do not overlap the slices and do not press the slices down onto the grill.
- This dish can be served cold or room temperature.

- To make this a Mediterranean-inspired breakfast, top with two sunny-side-up eggs and ½ cup hummus or cooked chickpeas.
- To enjoy as a lunch, pair with a serving of Garlic and Thyme Pressure Cooker Chicken (see page 169) and whole-grain pita bread.

- To have this as a delicious dinner, and to ensure you're Veggies Most, omit the pita bread from the lunch suggestion and have two to three servings of eggplant.

EGGPLANT

ROASTED EGGPLANT SPREAD
(Makes 4 servings, approx. ¼ cup each)

TOTAL TIME: **50 MINUTES** / PREP TIME: **10 MINUTES** / COOKING TIME: **40 MINUTES**

Parchment paper

Nonstick cooking spray

1   medium eggplant,
    sliced in half lengthwise

1½ tsp. tahini

1   clove garlic

1   Tbsp. fresh lemon juice

¼   tsp. ground cumin

2   Tbsp. chopped fresh
    parsley

Sea salt (or Himalayan
    salt) and ground
    black pepper (to taste;
    optional)

1. Preheat oven to 350° F.

2. Line a baking sheet with the parchment
   paper and lightly coat with cooking spray.

3. Place the eggplant on the baking sheet flat
   side down.

4. Bake 30 to 40 minutes, or until the eggplant
   is very soft and no longer holds its shape;
   set it aside to cool.

5. When the eggplant is cool enough to handle,
   use a spoon to scoop the flesh from the skin
   and place the flesh in a mesh strainer set
   over a bowl to drain; discard the skin.

6. Place the tahini, garlic, lemon juice and
   cumin in a food processor. Pulse until
   smooth, about six 1-second pulses.

7. Add the eggplant and the parsley to the
   tahini mixture; season with salt and pepper,
   if desired; pulse to combine, about three
   1-second pulses. Do not overprocess.

8. Transfer to a serving bowl. Serve immediately or store in an airtight container in the
   refrigerator up to 4 days.

Tips

■ Spread on sandwiches
and wraps, or serve as a
dip with veggies.

■ To make this a lunch,
pair it with a Spiced
Jumbo Burger (see page
173) placed on top of half
of a whole-grain bun or
wrap in a large lettuce leaf
and pair with a side of fruit.
Top the burger with 2
Tbsp. of the Roasted
Eggplant Spread and enjoy
the rest of the serving with
1 cup snackable veggies.

■ To make this a dinner,
omit the bun from the
lunch option and increase
your snackable veggie
serving to two cups.

PROTEIN

BAKED LEMON COD PACKETS
(Makes 1 serving)

TOTAL TIME: **12 MINUTES** / PREP TIME: **5 MINUTES** / COOKING TIME: **7 MINUTES**

Aluminum foil

Parchment paper

2   lemon slices, ¼-inch-thick rounds

2   fresh parsley sprigs

1   (4 oz.) raw cod fillet

1   dash garlic powder

Sea salt (or Himalayan salt) and ground black pepper (to taste; optional)

1. Preheat oven to 350° F; place a baking sheet in the oven to preheat.

2. Lay out a sheet of foil and top it with an equal size sheet of parchment paper.

3. Place 1 lemon slice in the center of the parchment paper. Top with 1 sprig of parsley. Place the cod on top of the lemon and parsley; season with the garlic powder and salt and pepper, if desired. Place the remaining slice of lemon and remaining sprig of parsley on top of the cod.

4. Fold up the edges of the parchment paper and foil around the cod; crimp it tightly to make a sealed packet.

5. Place the packet directly on the preheated sheet in the oven; bake for 7 minutes.

6. Carefully open the packet, being cautious to avoid rising steam. Discard the lemon and parsley; transfer the cod to a plate and serve immediately, or store refrigerated in an airtight container up to four days.

Tips

■ Try replacing the lemon and parsley with: chili, lime and cilantro; or garlic and thyme; or orange and rosemary.

■ To make this a delicious dinner, pair with one to two servings of Baked Zucchini Packets with Tomato and Herbs (see page 192).

■ You can buy frozen cod filets as a more budget-friendly option, and defrost them overnight in the refrigerator or a few hours prior to cooking.

■ The USDA recommends cooking fish to a safe minimum internal temperature of 145° F, as measured using a food thermometer.

■ To make this a filling lunch, pair with two servings of Greek Style Roasted Cauliflower (see page 158) and add ½ cup cooked chickpeas to the cauliflower mixture.

PROTEIN

CHEESY EGG WHITE, KALE & MUSHROOM PIZZA

(Makes 1 serving)

TOTAL TIME: **9 MINUTES** / PREP TIME: **5 MINUTES** / COOKING TIME: **4 MINUTES**

Nonstick cooking spray

4 large egg whites (½ cup)

¼ cup all-natural marinara sauce

2 Tbsp. shredded part-skim mozzarella cheese

¼ cup cooked chopped kale (optional)

¼ cup cooked sliced mushrooms (optional)

1. Heat a small skillet, lightly coated with cooking spray, over medium-high heat.

2. Add the egg whites to the skillet; do not stir. As the eggs set, lift the edges, letting the uncooked portion flow underneath; cook for 1 to 2 minutes, or until the eggs are set.

3. Spread the marinara sauce evenly over the top of the omelet. Top with the cheese, kale (if desired) and mushrooms (if desired); cook, covered, for 1 to 2 minutes, or until the cheese melts.

4. Cut into four slices; serve immediately.

Tips

- Serve with a salad or a veggie side.
- To make this a delicious breakfast, pair with a side of whole-grain toast.

- Substitute 1 large egg plus 2 large egg whites (¼ cup) for 4 large egg whites. Lightly beat them before adding to the skillet.
- To make this "breakfast for dinner" omit the whole-grain toast from the lunch suggestion and add more veggies.

- Top this with dried oregano, garlic powder or chili powder, if desired.
- To make this a satisfying lunch, pair with one to two servings of Spaghetti Squash Hash Browns (see page 187) and a side of whole-grain toast.

PROTEIN

CITRUS MARINATED TOFU

(Makes 3 servings, approx. ¾ cup each)

TOTAL TIME: **1 HOUR 25 MINUTES** / PREP TIME: **25 MINUTES** / COOKING TIME: **NONE**

1   (14-oz.) package extra firm tofu, drained, cut into 1-inch cubes

3   cloves garlic, finely chopped

2   Tbsp. fresh lime juice

1½ tsp. reduced-sodium soy sauce

½   tsp. ground coriander

½   tsp. sea salt (or Himalayan salt)

1. Place several layers of paper towels (or clean kitchen towels) on a cutting board (or baking sheet). Arrange the tofu cubes in a single layer on the towels; cover with several layers of paper towels (or clean kitchen towels).

2. Place another cutting board (or baking sheet) on top. Press the tofu for 20 minutes; weigh the board down with a heavy pot or cans of food.

3. While the tofu is being pressed, combine the garlic, lime juice, soy sauce, coriander and salt in a small mixing bowl.

4. Remove weights from the tofu and transfer the tofu to a small baking dish; pour the garlic mixture over the tofu. Cover tightly and marinate in refrigerator for 1 hour, up to overnight.

5. Divide evenly among three plates; serve immediately or store refrigerated in an airtight container up to five days.

Tips

■ To serve warm, cook in a medium nonstick skillet over medium-high heat until all sides are lightly browned, about 5 minutes.

■ The tofu can be eaten without additional cooking.

■ To make this a yummy lunch, pair it with the Quick and Easy Citrus Slaw (see page 154) and top it with one small orange.

■ Try adding marinated tofu and sliced green onions to miso soup.

■ To enjoy this for dinner, skip the orange from the lunch suggestion. If you're still hungry, have some snackable veggies so you can be dinner and done!

PROTEIN

CREAMY CHICKEN SALAD

(Makes 1 serving)

TOTAL TIME: **15 MINUTES** / PREP TIME: **15 MINUTES** / COOKING TIME: **NONE**

---

4   oz. cooked boneless, skinless chicken breast, chopped

1   small apple, chopped

2   stalks celery, chopped

2   Tbsp. reduced-fat (2%) plain Greek yogurt

2   Tbsp. fresh lemon juice

1   Tbsp. water

1   tsp. all-natural mayonnaise

3   cups chopped lettuce

Sea salt (or Himalayan salt) and ground black pepper (to taste; optional)

1. Combine the chicken, apple, celery, yogurt, lemon juice, water and mayonnaise in a medium bowl; mix well. Season with salt and pepper, if desired.

2. Place the lettuce in medium serving bowl; top with the chicken mixture.

Tips

■ You can swap the apple for ½ cup chopped grapes.

■ To enjoy this for lunch, pair with the Bacon and Date Cabbage Salad (see page 150) and wrap both salads in a whole-grain tortilla wrap.

■ To have this for dinner, omit the wrap from the lunch suggestion and have one to two servings of the Bacon and Date Cabbage Salad so you're full and satisfied and can be dinner and done!

PROTEIN

GARLIC & THYME
PRESSURE COOKER CHICKEN

(Makes 2 servings, 1 breast each)

TOTAL TIME: **15 MINUTES** / PREP TIME: **5 MINUTES** / COOKING TIME: **10 MINUTES**

1   stalk celery, cut in half

1   small carrot, chopped in half

¼   medium onion, sliced

2   (4-oz.) frozen chicken breasts, boneless, skinless

1   cup water

2   fresh thyme sprigs

2   cloves garlic, crushed

Sea salt (or Himalayan salt) and ground black pepper (to taste; optional)

1. Arrange the celery, carrot, and onion on bottom of an Instant Pot (or pressure cooker); arrange the frozen chicken on top of the vegetables.

2. Add the water; place the thyme and garlic on top of the chicken. Season with salt and pepper, if desired.

3. Seal the pot or cooker; cook on high, for 10 minutes. Release pressure manually or allow it to release naturally.

4. Transfer the chicken to a plate and serve immediately; discard the vegetables.

Tips

■ To make this recipe in a slow cooker, place all ingredients in the cooker and cook on low for 6 hours (use appliance in accordance with manufacturer's instructions).

■ The USDA recommends cooking poultry to a safe minimum internal temperature of 165° F, as measured using a food thermometer.

■ Make sure the frozen chicken pieces are not stuck together.

■ To make this a lunch, shred the chicken and add to Spaghetti Squash Taco Boats (see page 188) with ½ cup black beans.

■ To make this a dinner, shred the chicken and add to two to three servings of Spicy Peanut Sauce over Zoodles (see page 193).

> **PROTEIN**

LARA'S BAKED
SESAME SALMON

(Makes 1 serving)

TOTAL TIME: **23 MINUTES** / PREP TIME: **5 MINUTES** / COOKING TIME: **18 MINUTES**

1   (4-oz.) raw salmon fillet

Sea salt (or Himalayan salt) and ground black pepper (to taste; optional)

¼ tsp. sesame oil

¼ tsp. sesame seeds (white or black)

1. Preheat oven to 400° F.

2. Line a baking sheet with aluminum foil; place it in the oven to preheat.

3. Pat the salmon dry, then brush oil onto both sides of the salmon.

4. Carefully place the salmon, skin side down, on the preheated baking sheet; season with salt and pepper, if desired, and sprinkle with the sesame seeds. Bake for 18 minutes.

5. Transfer the salmon to a plate and serve immediately, or store refrigerated in an airtight container up to four days.

Tips

- To have as a delicious dinner, omit the corn from the lunch suggestion. If you need more veggies, add in a ½ serving of the Crispy Cabbage (see page 152).

- Try replacing the sesame seeds with everything bagel seasoning blend.

- The USDA recommends cooking fish to a safe minimum internal temperature of 145° F, as measured using a food thermometer.

- To enjoy as an Asian-inspired lunch, pair one serving with the Egg Roll in a Bowl (see page 153) and add ½ cup cooked corn to the egg roll recipe.

PROTEIN

PEANUT BUTTER & JELLY WONDER WHIP

(Makes 1 serving)

TOTAL TIME: **10 MINUTES** / PREP TIME: **10 MINUTES** / COOKING TIME: **NONE**

---

1 cup reduced-fat (2%) plain Greek yogurt

2 Tbsp. peanut butter powder

1 tsp. pure vanilla extract

Liquid stevia (to taste; optional)

Ground cinnamon (to taste; optional)

¼ cup fresh (or frozen) red grapes, cut in half

1. Combine the yogurt, peanut butter powder, vanilla extract, stevia (if desired) and cinnamon (if desired) in a serving bowl; mix well.

2. Top the yogurt mixture with grapes.

3. Serve immediately or store refrigerated in an airtight container for up to 1 day.

Tips

- For a delicious dinner, keep the grapes at ¼ cup and pair with two servings of the Quick and Easy Citrus Slaw (see page 154).

- Dry stevia can be substituted for liquid stevia.

- To enjoy as a breakfast, increase the grapes to ½ cup.

- For a simple sweet and savory mix-and-match lunch, increase the grapes to ½ cup and pair with a serving of Quick and Easy Citrus Slaw (see page 154).

PROTEIN

SLOW COOKER VEGGIES MOST & BEEF CHILI

(Makes 6 servings, approx. 2 cups each)

TOTAL TIME: **4 HOURS 25 MINUTES** / PREP TIME: **25 MINUTES** / COOKING TIME: **4 HOURS**

---

1   lb. raw 95% lean ground beef

2   cans (15 oz. each) kidney or pinto beans (or combination of both), drained, rinsed

1   (28-oz.) can diced tomatoes, no salt added

3   medium carrots, chopped

3   medium stalks celery, chopped

2   medium onions, chopped

1   medium red bell pepper, chopped

1   medium green bell pepper, chopped

5   cloves garlic, finely chopped

2   dried bay leaves

3   Tbsp. chili powder

1   Tbsp. dried oregano

1   Tbsp. ground cumin

1   Tbsp. ground smoked paprika

1   tsp. sea salt (or Himalayan salt)

½   tsp. ground coriander

¼   tsp. ground cayenne pepper (optional)

1. Combine the beef, beans and tomatoes with their juice in an 8-quart slow cooker; stir to mix.

2. Add the carrot, celery, onion, red and green bell peppers, garlic, bay leaves, chili powder, oregano, cumin, paprika, salt, coriander and cayenne pepper (if using); stir to mix.

3. Cook, covered, on high for 4 hours (or on low for 8 to 10 hours). Use the appliance in accordance with manufacturer's instructions.

4. Divide evenly between six serving bowls and serve immediately, or store refrigerated in an airtight container up to four days.

Tips

■ To make this a savory lunch, pair with two servings of Cauliflower Steaks with Red Pepper Sauce (see page 155) and add a ½ cup cooked corn to the chili.

■ To enjoy as a filling dinner, omit the corn from the lunch suggestion.

■ To make this recipe in an Instant Pot (note the order of ingredients differs slightly):

• Add the beans, tomatoes with their juice, bay leaves, chili powder, oregano, cumin, paprika, salt, coriander and cayenne pepper (if using); stir to combine.

• Add the carrots, celery, onion, red and green peppers and garlic; cook for 3 minutes or until softened.

• Turn the Instant Pot to the "chili/beans" setting and secure the lid on the pot. Cook for 20 minutes. Release the pressure manually or allow it to release naturally.

PROTEIN

SPICED JUMBO BURGER

(Makes 5 servings, 2 patties each)

TOTAL TIME: **41 MINUTES** / PREP TIME: **35 MINUTES** / COOKING TIME: **12 MINUTES**

Yogurt Sauce:

¼ cup reduced-fat (2%) plain Greek yogurt

¼ cup chopped fresh parsley

¼ cup chopped fresh mint

¼ cup finely chopped red bell pepper

¼ cup finely chopped shallot (or onion)

1 clove garlic, finely chopped

1 Tbsp. fresh lemon juice

Jumbo Burgers:

1 lb. raw 93% lean ground turkey

1 (14-oz.) bag frozen cauliflower rice, thawed, drained

3 Tbsp. finely chopped red bell pepper

3 Tbsp. finely chopped shallot (or onion)

1 tsp. ground cumin

1 tsp. chili powder

1 tsp. garlic powder

½ tsp. ground coriander

½ tsp. ground smoked paprika

Nonstick cooking spray

1. To make the yogurt sauce, combine the yogurt, parsley, mint, bell pepper, shallot (or onion), garlic and lemon juice in a medium bowl. Cover tightly and place in the refrigerator.

2. To make the jumbo burgers, combine the turkey, cauliflower, bell pepper, shallot (or onion), cumin, chili powder, garlic powder, coriander and paprika in a large mixing bowl; use clean hands to mix well.

3. Shape the turkey mixture into ten ½-inch-thick patties (approx. ¼ cup each); set aside.

4. Heat a medium nonstick skillet, lightly coated with cooking spray, over medium-high heat. Working in batches, add the patties to the skillet and cook for 2 to 3 minutes on each side, until lightly browned.

5. Serve two jumbo burgers topped with 2 Tbsp. yogurt sauce.

Tips

- If you prefer a dairy-free version, you can replace the yogurt sauce with the Roasted Eggplant Spread (see page 164) or a dairy-free accessory that you enjoy.

- To make this a lunch, pair it with ½ whole-grain bun and pair with two servings of Noah's Animal-Style Cauliflower (see page 159).

- To make this a dinner, chop up the burger and divide it evenly over two servings of the Eggplant Sandwich Thins (see page 162) and accessorize to your liking!

- You can substitute any extra-lean ground meat (beef, bison or a plant-based substitute) for the turkey.

- The USDA recommends cooking ground meat to a safe minimum internal temperature of 160° F, as measured using a food thermometer.

PROTEIN

TEMPEH BACON
(Makes 4 servings, approx. 5 pieces each)

TOTAL TIME: **1 HOUR 31 MINUTES** / PREP TIME: **6 MINUTES** / COOKING TIME: **25 MINUTES**

1   (8-oz.) package tempeh, sliced ¼-inch thick

2   Tbsp. reduced-sodium soy sauce

2   Tbsp. pure maple syrup

½   tsp. ground smoked paprika

½   tsp. sea salt (or Himalayan salt)

Nonstick cooking spray

1. Arrange the tempeh slices in a shallow baking dish; set aside.

2. Combine the soy sauce, maple syrup, paprika and salt in a small mixing bowl.

3. Pour the soy sauce mixture over the tempeh. Cover tightly and let it marinate in the refrigerator for at least 1 hour, or overnight.

4. Preheat oven to 350° F.

5. Line a baking sheet with parchment paper; lightly coat with cooking spray.

6. Arrange the tempeh on a baking sheet in a single layer. Bake for 20 to 25 minutes, turning halfway through, until browned.

Tips

- To enjoy as a breakfast, pair with a whole-grain English muffin and accessorize with avocado.

- Make this a yummy lunch by pairing it with a serving of Spaghetti Squash Hash Browns (see page 187) and a cup of bean-based soup.

- Enjoy for dinner by having the bacon with two to three servings of Spaghetti Squash Hash Browns.

SHAKEOLOGY

AÇAÍ POWER SHAKEOLOGY
(Makes 1 serving)

TOTAL TIME: **5 MINUTES** / PREP TIME: **5 MINUTES** / COOKING TIME: **NONE**

1 cup water

1 cup ice

1 scoop Vanilla Whey Shakeology (or Vanilla Plant-Based Vegan Shakeology)

1 cup baby spinach

½ (3.5-cz.) packet frozen unsweetened açaí puree

1 tsp. sunflower butter

1. Place the water, ice, Shakeology, spinach, açaí and sunflower butter in a blender; cover. Blend until smooth.

Tips

■ For a delectable dinner, make the shake as instructed and pair with one to two servings of Quick and Easy Citrus Slaw (see page 154).

■ To enjoy for breakfast, use the full açai puree packet to make sure you have an equal balance of protein (Shakeology) and FFCs (acai packet) so you are full, satisfied and fueled with energy to take on the day!

■ Take a tropical vacation during lunch by adding the full açai packet to the shake and pair it with Tropical Mango Salad (see page 201).

BIRTHDAY CAKE SHAKEOLOGY
(Makes 1 serving)

TOTAL TIME: **5 MINUTES** / PREP TIME: **5 MINUTES** / COOKING TIME: **NONE**

1	cup unsweetened almond milk
1	cup ice
1	scoop Vanilla Whey Shakeology
½	cup reduced-fat (2%) plain Greek yogurt
¼	large banana
1	tsp. pure birthday cake extract
½	tsp. edible plant-based sprinkles

1. Place the almond milk, ice, Shakeology, yogurt, banana and extract in a blender; cover. Blend until smooth.

2. Pour into a serving glass; garnish with the sprinkles.

Tips

- Substitute half a scoop of Vanilla Whey Shakeology and half a scoop of Strawberry Whey Shakeology for one scoop of Vanilla Whey Shakeology.

- To enjoy "cake" for breakfast, use ½ large banana (for your FFC) in the shake (which is your protein) to make this a sweet and satisfying Plate It! breakfast.

- Make your own healthier rainbow sprinkles with shredded coconut! Place 2 Tbsp. unsweetened shredded coconut in a resealable plastic bag, add 1 to 2 drops of all-natural food coloring; remove air from the bag, seal it, and shake until the coconut is evenly colored. Use any colors you like!

- Don't have pure birthday cake extract? Swap for ½ tsp. pure almond extract and ½ tsp. pure butter extract.

- Enjoy "cake" and pizza for lunch by using ½ large banana in the shake and pair it with one serving of Zucchini Pizza Coins (see page 195).

- For a pizza and "cake" dinner party, pair the shake (skip the banana) with one to two servings of Zucchini Pizza Coins.

CARROT CAKE SHAKEOLOGY
(Makes 1 serving)

TOTAL TIME: **5 MINUTES** / PREP TIME: **5 MINUTES** / COOKING TIME: **NONE**

1 cup unsweetened almond milk

1 cup ice

1 scoop Vanilla Whey Shakeology (or Vanilla Plant-Based Vegan Shakeology)

1 cup chopped or shredded carrots

1 Tbsp. hemp seeds

1 Tbsp. finely chopped orange peel (orange zest)

½ tsp. pure vanilla extract

1. Place the almond milk, ice, Shakeology, carrots, hemp seeds, orange peel and vanilla extract in a blender; cover. Blend until smooth.

Tips

■ For a super satisfying lunch, add ½ large orange to the recipe and pair with Kaitlin's Garlicky Carrots and Cauliflower Rice (see page 157).

■ To make this a complete breakfast, add ½ large orange to the shake so you have a balance of protein (coming from Shakeology) and FFCs (coming from the fruit). And the best part? You're getting "cake" and extra credit (from the carrots) at the start of your day!

■ To enjoy for dinner, start with Kaitlin's Garlicky Carrots and Cauliflower Rice and end with the Carrot Cake shake so you can easily be dinner and done, and you can find something fun and productive to do!

CHOCOLATE PEANUT BUTTER SHAKEOLOGY
(Makes 1 serving)

TOTAL TIME: **5 MINUTES** / PREP TIME: **5 MINUTES** / COOKING TIME: **NONE**

1 cup unsweetened almond milk

1 cup ice

1 scoop Chocolate Whey Shakeology (or Chocolate Plant-Based Vegan Shakeology)

½ cup frozen cauliflower rice

2 Tbsp. peanut butter powder

1. Place the almond milk, ice, Shakeology, cauliflower and peanut butter in a blender; cover. Blend until smooth.

Tips

■ For a simple and quick lunch, add ½ cup strawberries to the shake for your FFC and pair with Crispy Cabbage (see page 152) to make sure your meal is Veggies Most!

■ To make sure you get 50 percent protein and 50 percent FFCs for breakfast, add ½ large banana to the shake and start your day with chocolate, peanut butter, and banana goodness!

■ To make a satisfying dinner, make the shake as instructed above and pair with one to two servings of Eggplant Rollatini (see page 161). Enjoy the rollatini first, then have the shake; that way it feels like you're having dessert, but you're really just making it easier to be dinner and done!

SHAKEOLOGY

CHOCOLATE RASPBERRY TRUFFLE SHAKEOLOGY

(Makes 1 serving)

TOTAL TIME: **5 MINUTES** / PREP TIME: **5 MINUTES** / COOKING TIME: **NONE**

---

1 cup unsweetened almond milk

1 cup ice

1 scoop Chocolate Whey Shakeology (or Chocolate Plant-Based Vegan Shakeology)

¼ cup frozen raspberries

¼ tsp. pure vanilla or caramel extract (optional)

1. Place the almond milk, ice, Shakeology, raspberries and extract in a blender; cover. Blend until smooth.

Tips

■ To make this a Plate It! breakfast, increase the raspberries to ½ cup so you have an equal balance of protein and FFCs.

■ If you don't have raspberries, this recipe tastes great with other berries or a blend of whatever berries that you have on hand.

■ For a sweet and spicy lunch, increase the raspberries to ½ cup in the shake and pair with one serving Spicy Peanut Sauce over Zoodles (see page 193).

■ To have a sweet and savory Veggies Most dinner, make the shake as instructed and enjoy with one to two servings of Spaghetti Squash Carbonara (see page 186). Enjoy the shake after you've eaten your veggies so you can end the meal on a sweet and satisfying note!

CHOCOLATE SEA SALT SHAKEOLOGY

(Makes 1 serving)

TOTAL TIME: **5 MINUTES** / PREP TIME: **5 MINUTES** / COOKING TIME: **NONE**

---

1   cup unsweetened coco-
    nut milk beverage

1   cup ice

1   scoop Chocolate
    Whey Shakeology
    (or Chocolate
    Plant-Based Vegan
    Shakeology)

1   tsp. cacao nibs

1   dash sea salt
    (or Himalayan salt)

1. Place the coconut milk, ice, Shakeology and
   salt in a blender; cover. Blend until smooth.

Tips

■ To make this a satisfying
breakfast, add ½ large
banana to the blender.

■ For a "pizza and shake"
lunch, pair with one
serving of Eggplant
Pizzas (see page 160).

■ Enjoy a takeout-style
dinner by pairing the
shake with one to two
servings of Noah's
Animal Style Cauliflower
(see page 159).

SHAKEOLOGY

CREAMY COFFEE CAKE SHAKEOLOGY

(Makes 1 serving)

TOTAL TIME: **5 MINUTES** / PREP TIME: **5 MINUTES** / COOKING TIME: **NONE**

½ cup unsweetened almond milk

½ cup water

1 cup ice

1 scoop Café Latte Whey Shakeology (or Café Latte Plant-Based Vegan Shakeology)

¼ large banana

2 tsp. all-natural peanut butter

1. Place almond milk, water, ice, Shakeology, banana and peanut butter in a blender; cover. Blend until smooth.

Tips

■ To enjoy for dinner, make the recipe as instructed and pair with two to three servings of Three-Ingredient Spaghetti Squash Lasagna (see page 189).

■ To enjoy this shake as part of your breakfast, pair the shake (your protein) with a slice of whole-grain toast (which works as your FFC) and 1 Tbsp. all-natural peanut butter (your accessory).

■ For simple and satisfying lunch, increase the banana from ¼ to ½ so you have plenty of energy to get through the afternoon, and pair it with one serving of Cabbage Steaks with Creamy Ranch (see page 151).

SHAKEOLOGY

GINGERBREAD COOKIE SHAKEOLOGY
(Makes 1 serving)

TOTAL TIME: **5 MINUTES** / PREP TIME: **5 MINUTES** / COOKING TIME: **NONE**

1   cup unsweetened almond milk

1   cup ice

1   scoop Vanilla Whey Shakeology (or Vanilla Plant-Based Vegan Shakeology)

2   tsp. all-natural almond butter

¼   tsp. ground ginger

¼   tsp. ground clove

1. Place the almond milk, ice, Shakeology, almond butter, ginger and clove in a blender; cover. Blend until smooth.

Tips

■ For lunch, pair with one serving of Spaghetti Squash Taco Boats (so you're Veggies Most!) and add ½ cup cooked red or black beans to the squash mixture to help give you energy to conquer your afternoon!

■ To make this a filling breakfast, that can help fuel you for a powerful workout, pair the shake (your protein) with a toasted whole-grain English muffin (your FFC) topped with 1 Tbsp. all-natural almond butter (your accessory).

■ To enjoy a quick and easy dinner, pair the shake with the Kaitlin's Garlicky Carrots and Cauliflower Rice (see page 157). Enjoy the shake after you eat the veggie side so you're ending the meal with something sweet and satisfying, making it easier for you to ditch dessert and be dinner and done!

SHAKEOLOGY

GREEN MACHINE SHAKEOLOGY

(Makes 1 serving)

TOTAL TIME: **5 MINUTES** / PREP TIME: **5 MINUTES** / COOKING TIME: **NONE**

1 cup unsweetened coconut milk beverage

½ cup reduced-fat (2%) plain Greek yogurt

1 cup ice

1 scoop Vanilla Whey Shakeology

½ cup chopped raw kale (or spinach, or 1 scoop Shakeology Boost Power Greens)

½ cup frozen cauliflower rice

2 fresh basil leaves (optional)

1 dash finely chopped lime peel (lemon zest)

1. Place the coconut milk, yogurt, ice, Shakeology, kale, cauliflower, basil and lime zest in a blender; cover. Blend until smooth.

Tips

■ For a power-packed lunch, add ½ large green apple to the recipe and pair the shake with Crispy Cabbage (see page 152).

■ To enjoy for breakfast, add ½ large green apple to the recipe. With the protein from the Shakeology and Greek yogurt plus the stable energy coming from your FFC, the apple, this shake can help you feel fueled with all the right stuff to take on the day!

■ Make this a part of your dinner by keeping the recipe as is and pairing it with Cauliflower Steaks with Red Pepper Sauce (see page 155).

SHAKEOLOGY

TROPICAL POPSI-KALE SHAKEOLOGY
(Makes 1 serving)

TOTAL TIME: **5 MINUTES** / PREP TIME: **5 MINUTES** / COOKING TIME: **NONE**

1   cup unsweetened coconut milk beverage

1   cup ice

1   scoop Strawberry Whey Shakeology (or Tropical Strawberry Plant-Based Vegan Shakeology)

½   cup kale

¼   cup frozen pineapple

¼   cup frozen papaya (or orange or mango)

2   tsp. unsweetened shredded coconut

1. Place the coconut milk, ice, Shakeology, kale, pineapple, papaya (or orange or mango) and coconut in a blender; cover. Blend until smooth.

Tips

■ To make popsicles, omit the ice, then pour the blended smoothie into popsicle trays; freeze. Makes four snack(tional) servings.

■ Start your day with a tropical getaway by increasing the pineapple chunks to ½ cup so you have a good balance of the protein coming from Shakeology and the FFCs coming from the fruit, making this a Plate It! breakfast.

■ For a Veggies Most dinner, make the shake as instructed and pair with the Quick and Easy Citrus Slaw (see page 154).

■ To enjoy for lunch, increase the pineapple chunks to ½ cup in the shake and pair with the Quick and Easy Citrus Slaw.

KAITLIN'S SWEET & SAVORY SPAGHETTI SQUASH

(Makes 4 servings, approx. 1½ cups each)

TOTAL TIME: **50 MINUTES** / PREP TIME: **15 MINUTES** / COOKING TIME: **35 MINUTES**

Nonstick cooking spray

6 cups cooked spaghetti squash (see page 190)

1 Tbsp. olive oil

1 Tbsp. finely grated orange peel (orange zest)

1½ tsp. pure maple syrup

2 Tbsp. dried cranberries, finely chopped

2 Tbsp. walnuts, unsalted, chopped and toasted

1 clove garlic, finely chopped

1½ tsp. ground cinnamon

½ tsp. onion powder

1 dash ground clove

Sea salt (or Himalayan salt) or ground black pepper (to taste; optional)

1. Preheat oven to 350° F.

2. Lightly coat a 13 x 9-inch baking dish with cooking spray; set aside.

3. Combine the spaghetti squash, oil, orange peel, maple syrup, cranberries, walnuts, garlic, cinnamon, onion powder and clove in a large bowl. Season with salt and pepper, if desired.

4. Transfer the squash mixture to a prepared baking dish; bake for 25 to 35 minutes or until the squash starts to brown.

5. Divide evenly among four plates and serve immediately, or store refrigerated in an airtight container for up to four days.

Tips

- To make this a truly sweet and savory lunch, add ½ cup cubed cooked sweet potato to one serving of the squash mixture and pair it with Chocolate Sea Salt Shakeology (see page 180).

- To make this a simply satisfying dinner, skip the sweet potato in the lunch recommendation and just pair it with Chocolate Sea Salt Shakeology.

SPAGHETTI SQUASH

SPAGHETTI SQUASH CARBONARA
(Makes 4 servings, approx. 1 cup each)

TOTAL TIME: **14 MINUTES** / PREP TIME: **8 MINUTES** / COOKING TIME: **6 MINUTES**

Nonstick cooking spray

4   cups cooked spaghetti squash (see page 190)

½   cup low-sodium organic vegetable broth (or water), divided

1   large egg

2   large egg yolks

¼   cup finely grated Parmesan cheese

Sea salt (or Himalayan salt) and ground black pepper (to taste; optional)

1. Add the cooked spaghetti squash and ¼ cup broth (or water, if using) to a large nonstick skillet over medium heat; cook, covered, 3 to 5 minutes, stirring occasionally. Do not let the squash become dry.

2. As the squash cooks, heat the remaining ¼ cup of broth (or water, if using) in a small nonstick skillet or microwave for 1 minute; set aside.

3. When the squash is hot, remove the pan from the heat, then quickly perform the following two steps.

4. Whisk the egg and yolks in a medium bowl. Set the bowl on a kitchen towel to help prevent the bowl from sliding. Slowly drizzle the heated broth into the eggs, whisking constantly.

5. Immediately drizzle the egg mixture into the pan of heated spaghetti squash, stirring constantly. This will cook the egg mixture, making a creamy sauce.

6. Stir in the cheese; season with salt and pepper, if desired.

Tips

■ To make this a savory breakfast, top one serving of the carbonara with two sunny-side-up eggs and pair with a slice of whole-grain toast.

■ To enjoy for lunch, try adding Tempeh Bacon (see page 174) and ½ cup cooked peas to two servings of Spaghetti Squash Carbonara.

■ To enjoy for dinner, simply pair with Tempeh Bacon.

■ Pouring hot broth into eggs while whisking constantly will temper the eggs, to help make a smoother sauce, instead of scrambled eggs, when the egg mixture is added to hot food. For this recipe, it is okay if the sauce is not perfectly smooth; it will not affect the taste. Tempering eggs takes practice.

SPAGHETTI SQUASH HASH BROWNS

(Makes 4 servings, approx. 3 patties each)

TOTAL TIME: **52 MINUTES** / PREP TIME: **10 MINUTES** / COOKING TIME: **42 MINUTES**

Nonstick cooking spray

4 cups cooked spaghetti squash, divided (see page 190)

1 slice whole-grain (or whole wheat) bread

¼ cup green onion, thinly sliced (optional)

¾ cup red (or green) bell pepper, thinly sliced

Sea salt (or Himalayan salt) and ground black pepper (to taste; optional)

1. Preheat oven to 200° F.

2. Line a baking sheet with parchment paper; lightly coat with cooking spray. Set aside.

3. Place 1½ cups of squash and the bread in a food processor; pulse until smooth. Transfer to a large bowl.

4. Add the remaining 2½ cups of squash, the green onion (if using) and bell pepper to the squash puree; season with salt and pepper, if desired.

5. Heat a large nonstick skillet, lightly coated with cooking spray, over medium-high heat.

6. Working in batches, scoop ¼-cup portions of the squash mixture into the skillet and gently flatten; cook for 5 to 7 minutes, flip and cook 5 to 7 minutes more, until golden brown and crisp on both sides. If it browns too fast, reduce the heat as needed.

7. Transfer the hash brown patties to a baking sheet and keep them warm in the oven. Repeat until all the squash mixture is cooked.

8. Divide the hash brown patties evenly among four plates, or store refrigerated in an airtight container for up to four days.

Tips

■ To make this a yummy breakfast, pair with the Tempeh Bacon recipe (see page 174) or two over-easy eggs and enjoy with a cup of fresh fruit.

■ To ensure the hash browns cook evenly, do not overcrowd the skillet.

■ To enjoy as a lunch, top hash browns with the Creamy Chicken Salad recipe (see page 168) and pair with a bean-based soup.

■ Try cooking a single hash brown patty to test the skillet temperature before cooking the remaining patties.

■ To have this for dinner, swap the bean-based soup from the lunch suggestion for a broth-based veggie soup.

SPAGHETTI SQUASH TACO BOATS

(Makes 2 servings, 1 half squash each)

TOTAL TIME: **3 HOURS 3 MINUTES** / PREP TIME: **30 MINUTES** / COOKING TIME: **34 MINUTES**

Nonstick cooking spray

1 small spaghetti squash (approx. 2 lb.), whole, cooked (see page 190)

8 oz. mushrooms, chopped

1 medium carrot, chopped

1 medium onion, chopped

1 medium green bell pepper, chopped

½ cup water

1 (1-oz.) package low-sodium taco seasoning

1 tsp. dried oregano

1 small tomato, seeded, chopped (about 1 cup), divided

3 Tbsp. chopped fresh cilantro, divided

½ medium ripe avocado, chopped

2 Tbsp. fresh lime juice

2 Tbsp. shredded cheddar cheese

Tips

■ To have this as your dinner, have one Spaghetti Squash Taco Boat with one serving of the Slow Cooker Veggies Most and Beef Chili recipe.

1. Cut the cooked whole squash in half lengthwise. Remove the seeds and discard them. Scoop out the flesh of the squash and place it in a medium bowl; set aside. Reserve the skins.

2. Heat a large nonstick skillet, lightly coated with cooking spray, over medium-high heat.

3. Add the mushrooms and cook for 3 to 5 minutes, stirring frequently, until brown. Transfer to a medium bowl; set aside.

4. Add the carrot, onion and bell pepper to the skillet; cook for 3 to 5 minutes, stirring frequently, or until the onions are soft.

5. Return the mushrooms to the skillet. Add the water, taco seasoning and oregano; cook for 1 minute. Transfer the vegetable mixture to the bowl.

6. Add the spaghetti squash, ½ tomato and 2 Tbsp. cilantro; stir to combine.

7. Lightly coat a baking dish with cooking spray. Evenly divide the squash mixture between the reserved skins to make boats; place in the baking dish. Bake for 25 minutes or until the edges start to brown.

8. While the squash boats bake, combine the avocado, lime juice, remaining ½ tomato, and remaining 1 Tbsp. cilantro in a small bowl; set aside.

9. Top the squash boats evenly with the cheese; bake for 3 minutes or until the cheese melts.

10. Place the squash boats on two plates. Just before serving, top them evenly with the avocado mixture.

SPAGHETTI SQUASH

THREE-INGREDIENT SPAGHETTI SQUASH LASAGNA
(Makes 8 servings)

TOTAL TIME: **50 MINUTES** / PREP TIME: **10 MINUTES** / COOKING TIME: **40 MINUTES**

8   cups cooked spaghetti
    squash, divided (see
    page 190)
1   (25-oz.) jar all-natural
    marinara sauce, divided
2   cups part-skim ricotta
    cheese, divided
Aluminum foil

1. Preheat oven to 350° F.

2. Cover the bottom of a 13 x 9-inch baking dish with ⅓ jar of marinara. Cover the sauce with 4 cups squash; top evenly with 1 cup ricotta.

3. Spoon the second ⅓ jar of marinara evenly over the cheese. Cover evenly with the remaining 4 cups of squash. Spoon the remaining   jar of marinara evenly over the squash; top evenly with the remaining 1 cup of ricotta.

4. Cover with aluminum foil; bake for 40 minutes. Remove the foil for the last 10 minutes of cooking.

5. Cut the lasagna in 8 equal pieces and serve immediately, or store refrigerated in an airtight container for up to four days.

Tips

■ Try adding your own fillings to the middle layer (mushrooms, zucchini, eggplant, or spinach). Use this recipe as a starting point to make it your own.

■ To make this a lunch, pair one serving of Spiced Jumbo Burgers (see page 173) with two servings of the lasagna and pair with whole-grain garlic toast strips (simply use 2 tsp. butter and a sprinkle of garlic powder on top).

■ To make this a dinner, omit the garlic toast strips from the lunch recommendation.

Four Ways to Cook Spaghetti Squash

Spaghetti Squash is a versatile veggie, and so are the ways to cook it! Below are four different ways to make your squash based on the appliances and size of squash you have. No matter which method you go with, they all help you create the perfect base for the recipes on the preceding pages!

OVEN METHOD (WHOLE)

1. Preheat oven to 375° F.

2. Line a baking sheet with parchment paper and lightly coat it with cooking spray.

3. Pierce the spaghetti squash all over with the tip of a sharp knife.

4. Place the squash on the baking sheet; bake 45 to 90 minutes (see tips below), turning once, until it is soft and easily pierced with a knife in several places; set aside to cool until it can be handled comfortably, about 30 minutes.

5. When the squash is cool enough to handle, slice it in half lengthwise. Remove and discard the seeds. Use a spoon to scoop out the flesh.

OVEN METHOD (HALVES)

1. Preheat oven to 375 F.

2. Lightly coat a baking dish with cooking spray.

3. Carefully cut the spaghetti squash in half lengthwise. Remove and discard the seeds.

4. Arrange the squash flesh side down in a baking dish. Add water to cover the bottom of the dish to ½ inch.

5. Bake 30 to 45 minutes, until the squash is soft and easily pierced with a knife in several places. Set aside to cool until it can be handled comfortably; about 30 minutes.

6. When the squash is cool enough to handle, use a spoon to scoop out the flesh.

Tips

- These recipes can be made up to two days ahead of time and refrigerated in an airtight container for later use.

- Spaghetti squash come in many sizes:
  - Small (2 lbs.) yields approximately 2½ cups cooked squash.
  - Medium (4 lbs.) yields approximately 5 cups cooked squash.
  - Large (6 lbs.) yields approximately 8 cups cooked squash

- 1 (2-lb.) small spaghetti squash takes approximately 50 minutes to bake.
- 1 (4-lb.) medium spaghetti squash takes approximately 70 minutes to bake.
- 1 (6-lb.) large spaghetti squash takes approximately 90 minutes to bake.

PRESSURE COOKER METHOD (WHOLE)

1. Pierce the spaghetti squash all over with a knife.

2. Place a steamer insert into the pressure cooker and arrange the squash on the insert; add 1½ cups water.

3. Cook on high pressure for 15 minutes; quickly release the pressure when done (use appliance in accordance with manufacturer's instructions).

4. Check that the squash is soft and easily pierced with a knife in several places.

5. Set the squash aside to cool until it can be handled comfortably; about 30 minutes.

6. When the squash is cool enough to handle, slice it in half lengthwise. Remove and discard the seeds. Use a spoon to scoop out the flesh.

MICROWAVE METHOD (WHOLE)

1. Place the whole spaghetti squash in the microwave; cook, on high, for 3 minutes, or until it is tender enough to slice lengthwise.

2. Once the squash is sliced in half, use a spoon to remove the seeds from inside the spaghetti squash halves; discard the seeds.

3. Place both halves of the spaghetti squash in the microwave; cook, on high, for 6 to 8 minutes, or until you can easily remove spaghetti strands with a spoon. Place in a large bowl

- Do not microwave a whole spaghetti squash for more than 3 minutes. The squash could explode, damaging equipment and causing personal injury.
- Always use appliances in accordance with manufacturer's instructions.

- Spaghetti squash can get quite large and are hard to cut when raw. The Oven Method (whole) allows you to more easily handle and safely process the squash.

- A 6-quart pressure cooker can cook up to 1 (3-lb.) whole spaghetti squash.
- An 8-quart pressure cooker can cook up to 1 (4-lb.) whole spaghetti squash, or 2 (2-lb.) whole squash.

ZUCCHINI

BAKED ZUCCHINI PACKETS
with Tomato and Herbs
(Makes 2 servings, approx. 2 cups each)

TOTAL TIME: **25 MINUTES** / PREP TIME: **15 MINUTES** / COOKING TIME: **20 MINUTES**

---

2   medium zucchini,
    quartered lengthwise,
    sliced ¾-inch thick

2   medium tomatoes,
    chopped

2   cloves garlic, finely
    chopped

1½ tsp. dried Italian
    seasoning

2   tsp. olive oil

Sea salt (or Himalayan
    salt) and ground
    black pepper (to taste;
    optional)

Aluminum foil

1. Preheat oven to 400° F.

2. Place a baking sheet on the center rack.

3. Combine the zucchini, tomato, garlic, herbs
   and oil in a large bowl; season with salt and
   pepper, if desired.

4. Lay out two sheets of foil. Evenly divide the
   mixture between foil sheets; fold the edges
   of each tightly to create two sealed packets.

5. Place the foil packets directly onto the sheet
   in the oven. Cook for 20 to 25 minutes.
   Remove from the oven.

6. Allow the packets to cool slightly. Open
   carefully with tongs to avoid steam burns.

7. Transfer the contents to a serving dish.

Tips

■ After cooking, use tongs to
tear a hole in the packets
to allow the steam to
escape and avoid burns.

■ For a filling dinner, enjoy
one to two servings of
zucchini with a serving
of Slow Cooker Veggies
Most and Beef Chili (see
page 172).

■ This recipe can be cooked
on an outdoor grill. Turn
the packets over halfway
through cooking.

■ To enjoy for lunch, pair
one serving with a serving
of Slow Cooker Veggies
Most and Beef Chili and
add ½ cup cooked corn to
the chili.

ZUCCHINI

SPICY PEANUT SAUCE OVER ZOODLES

(Makes 2 servings, approx. 2 cups each)

TOTAL TIME: **28 MINUTES** / PREP TIME: **20 MINUTES** / COOKING TIME: **8 MINUTES**

Nonstick cooking spray

2 green onions, cut into 1-inch pieces

1 red bell pepper, thinly sliced

4 cloves garlic, finely chopped

½ tsp. crushed red pepper flakes (optional)

4 medium zucchini, spiralized

1 Tbsp. peanut butter powder

¼ tsp. ground ginger

1 tsp. reduced-sodium soy sauce

1 tsp. hot pepper sauce (like Sriracha)

½ tsp. rice wine vinegar

1 cup bean sprouts

1 Tbsp. peanuts, unsalted, chopped

¼ cup chopped fresh cilantro

1 lime, cut into wedges

1. Heat a large nonstick skillet over high heat; lightly coat with cooking spray.

2. Add the green onion and bell pepper; cook for 2 to 3 minutes, stirring frequently, until the vegetables start to soften.

3. Add the garlic and crushed red pepper flakes (if using); cook for 30 seconds, stirring frequently. Remove from the pan; set aside.

4. Add the zucchini, peanut powder, ginger, soy sauce, pepper sauce and vinegar to the same pan; cook for 2 to 4 minutes, stirring frequently.

5. Return the green onion mixture to the pan. Add the bean sprouts; gently fold to combine.

6. Evenly divide between two serving bowls; garnish evenly with peanuts, cilantro, and lime wedges.

Tips

■ A spiralizer is an inexpensive tool that cuts fresh veggies into noodles. You can use a spiralizer to cut the zucchini in this recipe.

■ If you don't have a spiralizer, using a vegetable peeler, cut each zucchini into lengthwise strips about ⅛-inch thick. Turn the zucchini slightly after cutting each strip to work evenly around the outside, stopping when you hit the seeds at the core. Discard the core. Cut the slices lengthwise into ½-inch ribbons.

■ For a yummy lunch, pair one serving zoodles with a serving of Garlic and Thyme Pressure Cooker Chicken (see page 169) and add ½ cup cooked lentils to the zoodles.

■ To make this a delicious dinner, pair one to two servings of zoodles with a serving of Garlic and Thyme Pressure Cooker Chicken.

ZUCCHINI

VEGGIES LOADED ZUCCHINI BOATS
(Makes 3 servings, 2 boats each)

TOTAL TIME: **50 MINUTES** / PREP TIME: **20 MINUTES** / COOKING TIME: **30 MINUTES**

Nonstick cooking spray

3   medium zucchini, cut in half lengthwise

¼   tsp. sea salt (or Himalayan salt)

1   small Chinese eggplant, chopped

8   oz. mushrooms, chopped

1   red bell pepper, chopped

4   cloves garlic, finely chopped

1   Tbsp. all-natural tomato paste

1   Tbsp. dried basil (or 3 Tbsp. fresh basil)

1   tsp. red wine vinegar

Sea salt (or Himalayan salt) and ground black pepper (to taste; optional)

2   Tbsp. pine nuts, chopped (optional)

2   Tbsp. grated Parmesan cheese

1. Preheat oven to 400° F with the rack in the middle position.

2. Lightly coat a baking dish with cooking spray; set aside.

3. Scoop out the inner flesh from the zucchini halves, using a spoon or melon baller. Chop the zucchini flesh and set it aside.

4. Place the zucchini halves in the baking dish, cut side up. Season with salt and pepper, if desired; set aside.

5. Heat a large nonstick skillet, lightly coated with cooking spray, over medium-high heat.

6. Add the zucchini flesh, eggplant, mushrooms, bell pepper and garlic; cook for 3 to 4 minutes, stirring frequently, or until water has been released and evaporated. Transfer to a bowl; set aside.

7. Add the tomato paste and basil to the same pan; cook for 1 minute, stirring frequently. Transfer to the bowl with the eggplant mixture.

8. Drizzle red wine vinegar over the eggplant mixture, season with salt and pepper, if desired; stir to combine.

9. Evenly spoon the eggplant mixture into the 6 zucchini halves. Top with the pine nuts, if desired, and the cheese.

10. Bake for 20 to 25 minutes, or until the zucchini are tender-crisp and the cheese is melted and lightly browned.

Tips

■ For a delicious and satisfying dinner, pair one to two servings with one Spiced Jumbo Burger.

ZUCCHINI

ZUCCHINI PIZZA COINS
(Makes 3 servings, approx. 5 each)

TOTAL TIME: **47 MINUTES** / PREP TIME: **20 MINUTES** / COOKING TIME: **27 MINUTES**

Parchment paper

Nonstick cooking spray

8 oz. sliced mushrooms

1 tsp. olive oil

¼ tsp. ground fennel seed

¼ tsp. ground smoked paprika

Sea salt (or Himalayan salt) and ground black pepper (to taste; optional)

3 medium zucchini, sliced ⅛-inch thick

1 (8-oz.) can all-natural tomato sauce

½ tsp. garlic powder

½ tsp. onion powder

1 tsp. dried Italian seasoning

½ cup finely shredded Italian cheese blend

2 Tbsp. fresh basil, sliced (or 2 tsp. dried basil)

1. Preheat oven to 400° F.

2. Line three baking sheets with the parchment paper (or work in batches); lightly coat with cooking spray. Set aside.

3. Combine the mushrooms, oil, fennel and paprika in a medium mixing bowl; season with salt and pepper, if desired.

4. Spread the mushroom mixture over one baking sheet. Bake for 10 minutes. Set aside to cool.

5. Arrange 5 zucchini slices in a circular, overlapping, rose-petal pattern on a prepared baking sheet. Repeat to make 15 individual clusters of "coins" to fill two baking sheets. Ensure there are no holes in the center of the clusters. Bake for 10 minutes; set aside.

6. Heat a small nonstick skillet over medium heat.

7. Add the tomato sauce, garlic powder and onion powder to the skillet; stir frequently until slightly thickened; set aside.

8. Carefully spoon the sauce over each cluster of zucchini "coins" (approx. 1 tsp. for each cluster). Evenly sprinkle the mushroom mixture over each cluster; top evenly with the cheese. Bake for 5 to 7 minutes, or until the cheese melts.

9. Garnish each cluster of "coins" with the basil.

Tips

■ For a pizza party dinner, pair one to two servings of pizza coins with a Cheesy Egg White, Kale and Mushroom Pizza.

■ Use a small amount of cooking spray on the baking sheets before lining with parchment paper to help keep the parchment paper from sliding.

■ To make this a pizza-licious lunch, pair one serving with a Cheesy Egg White, Kale and Mushroom Pizza (see page 166) and serve with a side of fresh fruit.

ZUCCHINI

ZUCCHINI NACHOS
(Makes 2 servings, approx. 2½ cups each)

TOTAL TIME: **55 MINUTES** / PREP TIME: **15 MINUTES** / COOKING TIME: **40 MINUTES**

Nonstick cooking spray

3 medium zucchini, sliced ⅛-inch thick

1 red bell pepper, chopped

1 small onion, chopped

8 oz. mushrooms, chopped

1 (1-oz.) package low-sodium taco seasoning

2 Tbsp. water

1 small tomato, chopped

½ cup grated cheddar cheese

½ cup jalapeños, pickled, sliced (optional)

Sea salt (or Himalayan salt) and ground black pepper (to taste; optional)

1. Heat oven to 425° F.

2. Line a baking sheet with the parchment paper; lightly coat with cooking spray.

3. Arrange the zucchini on the sheet in a single layer.

4. Bake for 20 to 25 minutes, or until the zucchini starts to brown on the edges. Remove from oven; set aside.

5. Heat a large nonstick skillet over medium-high heat; lightly coat with cooking spray.

6. Add the bell pepper and onion; cook for 5 minutes, stirring frequently. Transfer to a bowl; set aside.

7. Add the mushrooms to the same pan; cook for 3 to 4 minutes, stirring frequently.

8. Return the peppers and onions to the pan. Add the taco seasoning and water; cook for 1 minute, stirring frequently.

9. Evenly divide the mushroom mixture over the zucchini. Top with the tomato and cheese. Top with the jalapeño (if using).

10. Bake for 5 minutes or until the cheese melts.

11. Divide evenly between two plates, using a wide spatula; serve immediately, or store refrigerated in an airtight container for up to four days.

Tips

■ For a yummy "loaded nachos" lunch, top one serving of nachos with a serving of Slow Cooker Veggies Most and Beef Chili (see page 172) and add ½ cup cooked black beans to the chili.

■ If you don't want to use pre-packaged taco seasoning, try: ¾ Tbsp. chili powder, ¾ Tbsp. ground cumin, ½ Tbsp. ground paprika, ½ tsp. garlic powder, and ½ tsp. onion powder. Add salt to taste, if desired.

■ If the zucchini are small, use 4 to have enough slices to cover a baking sheet.

■ For a "nacho-average" delicious dinner, top one to two servings of nachos with a crumbled Spiced Jumbo Burger (see page 173).

BEACHBAR BREAKFAST BOWL
(Makes 1 serving)

TOTAL TIME: **5 MINUTES** / PREP TIME: **5 MINUTES** / COOKING TIME: **NONE**

¾ cup reduced-fat (2%) plain Greek yogurt

1 BEACHBAR, any flavor, chopped

1 cup strawberries, sliced

1. Add the yogurt to medium bowl; top with BEACHBAR and strawberries. Serve immediately.

Tips

■ This recipe is a great Plate It! breakfast.

■ To enjoy this for lunch, pair it with one serving Spaghetti Squash Hash Browns (see page 187).

■ To make this a dinner, omit the strawberries from the recipe and serve with two servings of Spaghetti Squash Hash Browns.

CHEESY CABBAGE STEAK TURKEY SANDWICH

(Makes 1 serving)

TOTAL TIME: **48 MINUTES** / PREP TIME: **10 MINUTES** / COOKING TIME: **38 MINUTES**

Parchment paper

Nonstick cooking spray

1   medium red cabbage

¼ tsp. ground paprika

¼ tsp. garlic powder

¼ tsp. onion powder

¼ tsp. ground cumin

6 oz. turkey deli slices (nitrate- and nitrite-free)

¼ cup shredded cheddar cheese

Aluminum foil

1. Preheat oven to 375° F. Line a baking sheet with the parchment paper and coat with the nonstick cooking spray.

2. To make the cabbage steaks, slice two 1½-inch-thick rounds from the center of a whole head of cabbage.

3. Place the cabbage steaks on the prepared baking sheet. Sprinkle them evenly with the paprika, garlic powder, onion powder and cumin. Bake for 15 to 20 minutes.

4. Top one cabbage steak with the turkey and cheese. Top it with the remaining cabbage steak.

5. Wrap the sandwich in aluminum foil and place the foil packet on the baking sheet. Place a weight or oven-safe pot or pan on top of the sandwich. Bake for 4 to 6 minutes.

Tips

■ To make with a panini press, wrap the sandwich in aluminum foil and place the foil packet in a preheated panini press. Press and cook until the cheese is melted, approximately 3 minutes.

■ Reserve the remaining cabbage for another meal, like the Cabbage Steaks with Creamy Ranch (see page 151).

■ This recipe is a great Plate It! dinner.

■ To make this a lunch option, pair it with your favorite FFC.

CHEESY TOMATO NOODLE SOUP

(Makes 4 servings, approx. 2 cups each)

TOTAL TIME: **15 MINUTES** / PREP TIME: **5 MINUTES** / COOKING TIME: **10 MINUTES**

1 (32 oz.) box prepared all-natural tomato soup

½ cup all-natural marinara sauce with basil

3 (8 oz.) bags tofu Shirataki noodles, drained (approx. 6 cups)

cup shredded part-skim mozzarella

1. Heat a large soup pot over medium heat. Add the soup and marinara sauce and bring to a gentle boil.

2. Add the noodles and cook for 2 minutes, stirring well to combine.

3. Divide the soup evenly between four bowls; top evenly with the cheese. Serve immediately.

Tips

■ Shirataki noodles can be found in many grocery stores and online.

■ Shirataki noodles may still contain water after draining, which may thin the soup a bit. If you prefer a thicker bisque, pat the noodles dry with paper towels before adding them to the pot.

■ To store the soup, allow it to cool at room temperature, then place it in a tightly covered container in the refrigerator for up to four days.

■ This recipe is a great veggie side.

■ To enjoy this for lunch, pair with one serving of Garlic and Thyme Pressure Cooker Chicken (see page 169) and add ½ cup black beans to the soup.

■ To make this a dinner, omit the black beans from the lunch suggestion.

SWEET & SAVORY EVERYTHING SAUCE

(Makes 5 servings, approx. 2 Tbsp. each)

TOTAL TIME: **3 MINUTES** / PREP TIME: **3 MINUTES** / COOKING TIME: **NONE**

½ cup carrot, chopped

1 clove garlic

1 tsp. ginger, peeled and finely chopped

3 Tbsp. tahini paste

2 Tbsp. white miso paste

2 Tbsp. rice vinegar

3 Tbsp. water

1 Tbsp. sesame oil

1 tsp. maple syrup

¼ tsp. ground black pepper

1. Place the carrot, garlic, ginger, tahini, miso, vinegar, water, sesame oil, maple syrup and pepper in a blender; cover. Blend until very smooth. Add more water if needed.

2. Serve immediately, or store refrigerated in an airtight container for up to five days.

Tips

■ Use this sauce on everything from roasted vegetables to salads, fish and poultry, spread on sandwiches, or use as a dip for raw veggies.

■ The sauce may thicken in the refrigerator. Set it out at room temperature for 15 to 20 minutes before serving; if needed, stir in more water, one teaspoon at a time, until the sauce reaches the desired consistency.

■ This recipe is a perfect accessory. Pair it with any veggie side in this book!

THE MINDSET MEMBERSHIP RECIPES

TROPICAL MANGO SALAD

(Makes 2 servings)

TOTAL TIME: **17 MINUTES** / PREP TIME: **15 MINUTES** / COOKING TIME: **2 MINUTES**

2 Tbsp. unsweetened shredded coconut

1 clove garlic, finely chopped

2 Tbsp. 100% orange juice (or ½ orange, squeezed)

1 tsp. olive oil

1 tsp. mustard

1 tsp. honey

Sea salt (or Himalayan salt) and ground black pepper (to taste; optional)

2 heads lettuce, chopped

1 medium mango, peeled and chopped

½ red bell pepper, chopped

½ orange bell pepper, chopped

½ yellow bell pepper, chopped

½ red onion, chopped

¼ cup chopped fresh cilantro

¼ medium ripe avocado, sliced

1. Heat a small pan over medium heat; add the coconut. Stir frequently for 2 minutes, or until the coconut is fragrant and toasted; remove from the pan and set aside.

2. To make the dressing, combine the garlic, orange juice, oil, mustard, honey, salt and pepper, if desired, in a small mixing bowl; whisk to blend. Set aside.

3. Combine the lettuce, mango, red pepper, orange pepper, yellow pepper, onion and cilantro in a large bowl; drizzle with the dressing and toss gently to coat. Top with the avocado and coconut. Divide evenly between two medium bowls.

Tips

- This recipe is a perfect veggie side.

- To enjoy for lunch, pair with one serving of Citrus Marinated Tofu (see page 167) and top with a small orange.

- To have this for dinner, omit the orange from the recommended lunch option.

NEVER
SAY "NO"
TO EATING

Kiss Deprivation Goodbye
Using These Simple Strategies.

"YOU CAN'T HAVE THAT."

You'll never hear those words from my mouth. I never want you to say "no" to eating unless you're feeling very focused and being offered something that isn't worth it, and it's followed by "Thanks, I'm good for now." In fact, whatever you do, make sure you aren't feeling deprived! Deprivation backfires badly and leads to long-term misery, not results. So instead of worrying about what not to eat, we'll take time in this chapter to think about how to eat *more*, and more positively, using two strategies that will help you do just that:

- *The More? Sure! Model*

- *The Push Off Method, aka Delay, Don't Deny*

Each one is simple to learn and, with time and practice, will build long-lasting weight-loss habits that will become second nature. Ready to learn more? Sure!

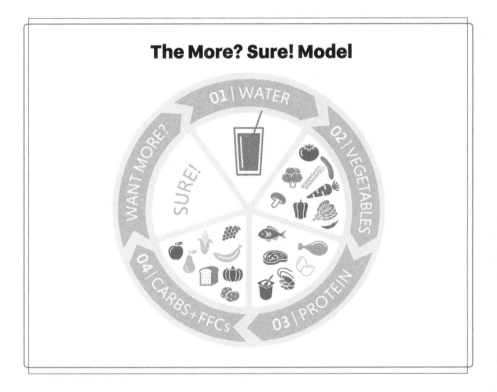

The More? Sure! Model

01 | WATER
02 | VEGETABLES
03 | PROTEIN
04 | CARBS+FFCs
WANT MORE?
SURE!

SIDE FROM MY beautiful children, my More? Sure! model is my most brilliant creation to date, and I use it literally every day. It is the greatest tool—specifically for someone with a big appetite (e.g., me) or for anyone who frequents social events, restaurants and family-style meals. Whenever you're faced with lots of food options, you'll simply follow the steps to help you stay in control.

Always be sure to start at the top of the cycle with Water First, especially when you have a long eating window ahead, like a weekend afternoon at Mom's house or a wedding, and you really want to pace yourself with the food. Follow the water with veggies, because as you surely remember, we always want veggies to be the first bite and what we fill up on, which is even more essential if you're surrounded by more food and temptations than usual. Next, choose and eat your protein, because that kicks in your sense of fullness to prevent unnecessary overeating and boost your overall sense of control. Then, if you want an FFC or silly treat, you'll be much more selective and in control.

If a spoonful of those crispy smashed potatoes turns out to be more delicious and tempting than you anticipated and you want More? Sure! Just go back around the circle again, starting with a nice big glass of water, sparkling water or unsweetened iced tea. Chances are, once you go around again, you'll be so fully satisfied that you don't even need the extra silly treat—or if you do, it will be *one* additional serving rather than multiple, like in the past. That's why, with the More? Sure! model, you're never saying no to eating. You're simply approaching it in a way that contributes to positive weight loss.

Some eating events, like weekend barbecues, can completely throw you off if you walk in hungry and without the More? Sure! model in your toolkit. If you start with a cocktail, chips and dip, and fried appetizers, you could easily eat 1,000 calories before the meat gets off the grill. Yet, with the More? Sure! model, you'll always be more in line and on track. Here's how that barbecue could go using it:

- You'll walk in and be sure to bypass the booze and chips. Instead, you'll immediately pour yourself a large cup of Water First. (If you want to be ahead of the game, you'll bring your own 2B Mindset water bottle and go straight to filling it up.)

- Next, you'll focus on finding veggies. If you didn't gift your hostess a veggie platter (great idea!), then find a salad or baby carrots and celery that may be hiding near the buffalo wings, to lightly dip in some ranch. Once you've snacked on at least one or two fistfuls of that, you can think about the protein.

- At this point, more options are likely off the grill. You can decide if you can split the sausage with a friend and pair it with some chicken breast or a drumstick, or opt for lean steak. If you decide you want a burger instead, rethink the bun if you start eyeing that cocktail, corn on the cob or fresh watermelon with greater appeal in the moment. When your choices take this route, every part of you feels more comfortable and empowered. This way you can finally see how fun it is to be in Weight Loss Mode without compromising your social life.

Or let's say it's the end of a long day, and you want to skip making dinner, preferring to go straight for the pretzels in the pantry. Before you do, first start on top of the circle and find your way around before testing yourself with that salty bag of refined carbs. You are essentially pushing off the most addictive foods to the point when you can control them rather than falling back into the rut of having them control you. While you may think that you can't be trusted with carbs altogether, you will really impress yourself with the level of "balanced" eating you can create by using this method. It's a life-changing system that becomes muscle memory the more you use it. It gets you to a magical place, along with the 2 Bunnies, where you can finally view food as purposeful and be free of your deeper emotional relationship with it.

HOW TO TELL IF YOU'RE ACTUALLY HUNGRY

THE MORE? SURE! MODEL is a foolproof way to never say no to eating. However, before using it, it's important to *ask yourself if you're actually hungry for more food,* and if so, why? This context will help you make the best choice in the moment, and in the future.

Here are three quick questions to run by yourself when the desire for more food strikes:

Am I Eating Enough at Meals?

You might be hungry because you're not eating enough at mealtime. It'll feel weird at first, maybe even a little wrong, you know, actually *eating* on a weight-loss plan. But I want you to feel full. Don't be afraid of eating multiple servings of those cauliflower steaks, eggplant pizzas or a second cheesy kale and mushroom pizza. Weight gain does not come from a really big, satisfying meal of veggies and protein. It comes from not eating enough at a meal and then being vulnerable to temptations, cravings and mindless snacking later as a result.

Everyone's different, but I recommend increasing your protein serving, not skipping meals, and eating raw veggies whenever you want, as long as you're also drinking Water First. Never be scared to add more veggies and more proteins to your dinner so you can be "dinner and done." If I've had a light dinner, such as a small kale salmon salad, and still feel like I'm a bit hungry and want something sweet, I'll blend ⅔–¾ cup of water with a cup of cauliflower rice, a cup of ice and a scoop of chocolate Shakeology. If it's an extra sweet craving (darn you, PMS!), I may even add some cinnamon and vanilla extract to make it feel more indulgent. My trick is to use less liquid than usual so it's thick like ice cream, pour it in a large bowl, and eat it with a spoon. It's a perfect under-200-calorie treat that's packed with water, veggies, superfoods, and additional protein that takes the hunger edge off and still helps me lose weight.

Loading up can be a good thing. For example, one of my clients, Kaitlin, told me she always got hungry after her breakfast of scrambled egg whites and a whole-grain English muffin. Well, sure, if you're just eating protein and an FFC, you might be hungry mid-morning. I told her to try drinking more water, add in veggies like spinach and mushrooms, and not be afraid to accessorize with some turkey bacon or cheese. That way, she'd find that she stayed fuller longer. After she did that, she not only felt satisfied until lunch, she also started losing more weight!

Also, don't be afraid to add a minestrone soup to your dinner, or to add a couple of cabbage steaks (that's simply sliced cabbage, sprayed with olive oil and baked until tender on the inside and crispy on the edges). One member told me she wanted to eat a whole bag of cauliflower rice but was nervous it would be too much—so I said, try it and see. I almost always eat a whole 14-ounce bag at a time. And if you're still hungry after that, refer to the More? Sure! Model. You can eat, enjoy and move on, and then your mindset is clear to focus on other things so you never feel hung up on food.

By the way, not eating enough food can hinder your weight loss (like it did for my client)—if you're not eating enough of the right things. If all you're eating is, say, a handful of crackers here and a handful of dried fruit there, you might get through the day, but you'll feel hungry and distracted because you're never really full. You can eat more and weigh less if you eat more of the right things.

Is It Habit or Hunger?

Sheena F., a 2B Mindset devotee, asked me once if she could have multiple snacks throughout the day. The best answer for those kinds of questions is to try it, track it and see. But you have to ask yourself why you need more snacks. Is it habit or is it hunger? Are you "hungry" because time has passed, and you're used to feeding yourself at nine p.m.? Or is it because you're *actually* hungry? And if you're not actually hungry, you always have to ask yourself: Why am I eating? Are you bored? Are you tired?? And if you *are* hungry, ask: What *should* I be eating? Look to the More? Sure! Model for the answer. You should also analyze your tracker, be honest and ask yourself: Am I "veggies some" or am I truly Veggies Most? Am I not eating enough protein at each meal? Do I need to go food shopping or experiment with some new healthy recipes? Also look at the times you're eating; this can help give you insight into what changes you need to make to see greater success with your weight loss.

Do I Need this Eating Opportunity (DINTEO)?

I'm going to repeat this question until it becomes second nature for you. It's one of the biggest differences between your old mindset and new mindset. Eating opportunities pop up constantly (free pastries when getting coffee, cookies on the counter, breadbasket lingering on the table, etc.), but when they do, ask yourself, *"Do I need this eating opportunity?"* Chances are, the answer is "No!" because so often this happens when you're not even feeling hungry. And even if you are hungry, the foods you're encountering are not typically the ones that you want to eat to satisfy your hunger. These are usually the foods that take you on a backward route on the More? Sure! Model. (Let's call it the Weight Gain Model.)

You may be so used to eating seven times a day, and not even realizing it, just grabbing a handful of trail mix or cereal from the counter or a white minty circle from the candy dish. Asking yourself DINTEO doesn't deprive you, it empowers you! You're not saying, "I can't have it." You're simply bringing a sense of awareness and independence to your decision, rather than being a passive puppet controlled by your environment. I was recently in a doctor's office and was tempted by a bowl of chocolates (ironic, huh?). I was a centimeter away from grabbing a golden wrapper (without even thinking) when I remembered DINTEO!, chuckled a solid, "Not at all!" in my mind, and grabbed a magazine instead. In these cases, if the food wasn't there, you would likely never think to eat it. Eating just because it's in sight and therefore in stomach is not only what makes us accumulate so many pounds unconsciously, but it's ultimately what has made you feel so powerless about food. If you decide that yes, you do want the food, then fully enjoy it, track it and move on.

Ilana—ism

If You Nibble it, Scribble It.

Over time with consistent tracking, DINTEO will become second nature and you'll become the "mindful" eater you've always dreamed 2B.

Write "DINTEO" on a sticky note and put it on that shelf of the pantry where you need it the most. This will help you reinforce the mindset and stay more focused on your plan. If this all feels like something you could never see yourself doing consistently, remember everything in this book becomes easier and more fun with time. I know I am throwing a lot of suggestions at you. The first few weeks are the most challenging, because you're developing these suggestions as new habits. After brushing your teeth, you'll think, *I need to get on the scale...* when you were pretending to avoid it before. Before you sip your coffee, you'll remember, "I need to drink Water First." In the car, you may want to stop for something silly, but instead you'll say, "Let me pull these veggies out of my bag." After you put away dinner, rather than reaching for the remote, you'll reach for your tracking device to write down what you ate. The more you practice these habits, the more effortless they become. You never have to be "perfect," and in fact, there is no "perfect" way to follow the program, but the more driven you are to instill these habits in your life, the better and longer lasting your results will be. This includes asking yourself "DINTEO?" Think about it: You didn't learn how to ride a bike or swim in one day, and you don't learn them solely by reading about them in a book. These skills take time, consistent practice and patience with yourself until they become effortless.

And don't forget 2B Mindset is flexible enough to revolve around your hunger. You'll hear me tell you not to skip meals, but if skipping breakfast works for your weight loss, it works for you. A 2B Mindsetter named Sherry told me she's not hungry first thing in the morning, especially after drinking so much Water First. She gets up at 6:45 a.m. and she doesn't eat until 9:45 a.m. That's okay. You don't have to force yourself to eat if you're not hungry.

I just want to make sure that when you are ready to eat, you approach it with the More? Sure! model and Plate It! method in mind. No matter what you eat or how it goes, track it and use the scale to make sure you create a system of strategies that supports you—like the ones described in this chapter!

2B MINDSET SUCCESS STORY

*Sabrina H., an Independent Team Beachbody Coach, 31, Pierrefonds, Quebec, Canada,
lost 58.4 pounds in 16 months**

"I was so tired and scared because I lost control of my body."

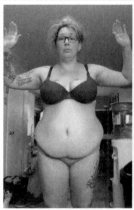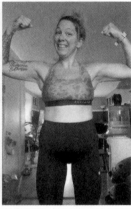

**Results vary depending on starting point and effort
and following Beachbody fitness programs.*

YOU DON'T HAVE to starve yourself to lose weight—something Sabrina H. didn't understand until she discovered the 2B Mindset. During her third pregnancy, Sabrina gained 70 pounds with her weight plateauing at 256 pounds. "I was so tired and scared because I lost control of my body," she confesses. In the past, her go-to method for losing weight was starvation. However, once she watched my 2B Mindset videos, she realized that food wasn't the enemy. "I realized that food is to fuel our body!" she explains. "My relationship with food went from an 'If I eat I won't lose, so I will starve myself' diet to huge plates of colorful veggies. So much food!" Her relationship with the scale also changed dramatically. "I use it now as a tool to know what my body likes and does not like!" she says. "Ilana gave me faith that I could do this! Four simple rules, I did it and every day I keep pushing play and dialing in my nutrition," she says. Sabrina plans on using the 2B Mindset for life. "Not because I *have* to, because I want to," she attests. "I feel healthy and feel like me!"

THE PUSH OFF METHOD, AKA DELAY, DON'T DENY

AS YOU KNOW by now, with 2B Mindset, you never need to say no to eating. But sometimes you might choose to say, "Not yet." This relates in particular to silly treats, holidays like Halloween, vacations or functions where you face an excessive amount of eating and treating opportunities. The idea is that you "push off" the eating opportunity until a later time, like a date night, so it stays special. The anticipation of delayed gratification, you'll soon realize, actually heightens your self-confidence and the sensory experience when you eventually do partake in a treat. You're simply delaying it, not denying it.

After all, it's not going anywhere.

Let's look at a real-life scenario to illustrate this. One Friday, Connie, who follows the 2B Mindset, told me she had an Italian wedding to go to that weekend. "There'll be a five-course meal," she said. "Any advice? Should I skip all the hors d'oeuvres and go straight to the main entree?"

Try the Push Off Method, I told her.

Five courses is probably three to five times more food than you need (or even want to have) at a meal. It's not that you shouldn't eat at the dinner, but do you need to eat and clear all five plates? Nah (and your dress would agree, too). Perhaps you eat every other course, or dance through one, or hold a tea during one, or visit the bride or another table during one. There's a lot of food at weddings, but don't make it all about food. Check out the flower arrangements. Meet someone from the other side. Enter the photo booth. Dance. Wish the couple well. Enjoy the *whole* wedding. Push off the food. And when you do eat, be present: Sit, look, taste the crumbs, taste the enjoyment. Just don't forget to look up and be social.

And sometimes, it makes sense to pregame! I like to go into long weddings or other eating opportunities after I've already met my water goal for the day and had a quick vegetable omelet or a

Shakeology with a lot of greens mixed in. If you're somewhat full and clear-headed, you won't spend the whole Electric Slide gliding up and down the buffet table.

You can use the Push Off Method not just at big events, but every day. Instead of swinging by your favorite bakery on your way home from work because someone wouldn't stop talking about the pastries you love, tell yourself, "I don't need them right now, it's just Tuesday. I will plan to have them at an upcoming special occasion." If you take care of a kid under 15, there's a good chance you see pizza at least once a week. Between birthday parties, school events and playdates, you are likely seeing the same semi-cold, nothing-special pie in similarly loud and distracting scenarios. Even if the pizza looks particularly good, remind yourself that there will always be pizza and plan to go home later and defrost some veggies to top with melted cheese, oregano,

---

Ilana-ism

Weight Loss Is a Treat

Next time you are feeling overworked, in a slump and deserving of a treat, remind yourself of the countless treats involved in weight loss: better health, energy, physical capability, wardrobe possibilities, greater self-confidence and a less stressed mind. This will help you turn to a more productive treat that can help your progress, such as taking a bath and getting to bed early, planning a trip for the future that will help keep you motivated to keep going, or cutting up the veggies in the fridge to assemble veggie bags in preparation for your days ahead. And when you've decided you're Dinner and Done and someone nearby is tempting you with a bowl of snacks, remind yourself that if you really want them, you can have them tomorrow morning.

garlic powder and chili flakes for a more intentional—and maybe even tastier—experience. Make a plan to push it off until you're at some special pizza place that you've been looking forward to trying, a place where you can actually focus on how it tastes and not on the boogers flying out of kids' noses. Then focus on what your body needs—water, veggies, a nice walk.

When it comes time for that special occasion, enjoy it, track it and move on. Or you may not even want it because you're having great success with your weight loss, and sticking with it is more satisfying than a piece of pizza like the ones you've had countless times earlier in your life.

You will learn so much from practicing the Push Off Method. Here are three common benefits of putting it into practice:

- *You will find that the more selective you become—and the more time that elapses between indulgences—the more enjoyable the treat.* We all know that fries taste better when you're in a better state, so save that special opportunity until you've hit your goal weight and are confident in maintaining it. That will strip away any potential feelings of guilt and lead to immense satisfaction.

- *You might want to push old faves—off a cliff.* Once you've been accustomed to eating better-for-you foods and enjoying the wonderful treat of weight loss, you may take a bite of cheese curls, your old favorite, and wonder how you ever had a taste for such an artificial flavor. This shocking revelation has happened to me with too many foods to count—from chocolate kisses, which taste nothing like real 70 percent-
plus chocolate to packaged gummies that feel so sticky and overly sweet I can almost feel my bloodstream form into syrup.

- *You will be reminded how harmful these foods can be for your body and mindset.* You may feel like you've put in your time with eating veggies, and it's time to treat yourself to some of your kid's or coworkers' snacks. What starts with chocolate-covered pretzels soon

The Push Off Method on Vacation

On vacation the temptations accelerate throughout the day. You want gelato after lunch, a cocktail for happy hour and the special cuisine wherever you are. I've worked with dozens of people pre- and post-vacation, and I promise if you come back to a large and unnecessary weight gain, it can dampen your memories and perceived experience of the trip; it's not worth it. You want your vacations filled with good energy for activities, confidence to take pictures and wear what you want. You want to bring your attention to other guiltless indulgences that enhance your experience, like walking through art galleries, attending a concert, taking a boat ride or bike tour or catching the sunset. You want to plan what you eat around the activities you want to do, not plan activities around what and where you want to eat. So before you plan another foodie-focused trip with a list of restaurant destinations, consider these next tips:

- *I recommend never dropping the ball first thing in the morning.* If you start a vacation day with a hefty stack of pancakes and syrup, you are going to set your whole day up for lethargy and increased carb cravings that can turn a simple trip into a five-pound weight gain. Begin your day with a breakfast you might have at home—a veggie omelet, whole-grain toast, etc.—instead of a chocolate crepe the size of a hubcap.

- *For a multiday trip, make your first day a solid, lean day to set the tone of the trip*—then add one special thing, like a glass of wine or a delicious plate of pasta, for each day that follows.

- *Don't leave home unless you have—at the very least—your tracker and water bottle.* Even just seeing them float around your hotel room, handbag or backpack will remind you of your mindset, your goals and where you truly want 2B.

turns into handfuls of chocolate chips, stale crackers and half a block of cheese. After a momentary feeling of frustration and defeat, you'll track it and reinforce how much better you feel when you're following the plan rather than deviating from it. This will become a powerful learning experience for you and teach you what's worth pushing off for later and what's simply not worth your time.

CHAPTER SUMMARY

- *If you're still hungry, follow the More? Sure! model: 1) Drink water, then 2) eat vegetables, then 3) enjoy some protein and then 4) have some FFCs and then—still hungry? Start the cycle over.*

- *If you find yourself hungry often, ask yourself if you're eating enough at mealtimes, if you are eating out of habit and DINTEO (Do I Need This Eating Opportunity?).*

- *The Push Off Method means you "push off" the eating opportunity until a later time, like a date night, so that it stays special.*

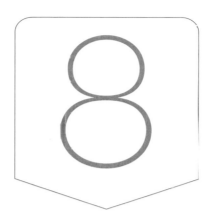

OLD MINDSET/ NEW MINDSET

Flip the Switch to Get Free of the Past and Enter Your New Future.

IF YOU'RE PERPETUALLY overweight, struggle with emotional or mindless eating, or lose weight only to see it come right back on, chances are it's not just your body but your mind that needs a change. I want your choices to come from empowerment and enjoyment, not deprivation and despair. That is the power of the 2B Mindset and essential to its proven sustainable success.

A good day begins with a good mindset; I've seen it proven time and again.

For example, take Shelly, who did the 2B Mindset online, then later came to see me as a client. Shelly recently told me about her late-night cravings and how she couldn't control them. She did the plan and then gained the weight back after a summer trip, which led to a self-sabotaging spiral. "I'm running a business," Shelly told me, "and can't find anyone to help me." She was jealous of SAHMs—stay-at-home moms—who drop their kids off and go work out. "It's so much easier for them to keep the weight off," she complained, "and there's no time between pickup and dropoff to do anything but work!"

A week later, she had turned completely around. You know why? I asked her to just focus on drinking one bottle of water on her way to the office and eating two cups of veggies by two p.m. I kept it simple. I didn't want to add more to her busy life.

Shelly got it together, had no cravings and lost four pounds.

She ultimately said she couldn't stand to listen to herself complain. "I run my own business," she remembered. "I am my own boss. Who am I to say I don't have the time to work out?" She took the time to go on an outdoor hike—and all of her late-night cravings? They vanished. Gone. Because she dropped the excuses, put on her boss lady pants and took control.

The late-night cravings didn't magically disappear because she felt full and satisfied; it happened because she became filled up with joy, energy, independence and relief. She's also proof that exercise is not only helpful for weight loss because it burns calories, but also because it allows you time to concentrate on yourself—your life, your body, your goals—and it makes everything feel more enjoyable.

Shelly got out of the past and into the future. Now it's your turn. Let my Ilana-isms guide you there.

THE NEW MINDSETS

OLD MINDSET: *I Will Never Lose All This Weight*
NEW MINDSET: *I Can Do Anything,*
        Focus on Two Pounds at a Time

Two pounds. That's all you have to lose. And then another two. And then another two. Look at each two pounds as a game for you to win. Rather than feeling you have to push a boulder up a mountain, inch it up. Not every day is going to be a weight-loss day at first. But every tip and strategy you learn in this book—and in the videos online—will help you unlock the next two pounds. And the next.

You need to look at this as a pacing thing. The 2B Mindset isn't a short burst of exercise, especially if you have 30 or more pounds to lose. You will need endurance and a forward-thinking mindset and you can do it. This is something you will do long term and be able and want to do long term. Every bit of effort you put in will make it more effortless to sustain, so the result is all worth your time and energy. Instead of worrying so much about losing "all this weight," be appreciative of the fact that you have a great system this time that works for you, and every day you are getting healthier and happier than the day before. You are progressing, and that's what is important. You are eating better, feeling better and are more empowered each day. You want the number on the scale to go down, sure, but you also need to recognize the positive changes you're making for your mental and physical health at the same time. Are you feeling more confident and making better choices? If so, then you will be happy *as* you drop the weight, not just *once* you drop the weight.

OLD MINDSET: *I Gained Weight and I Feel Gross*
NEW MINDSET: *I am Making Progress and I Can Drop It*

Feeling "gross" propels self-sabotage and negativity. Feeling like you can lose it propels self-confidence and productivity.

I know about feeling gross. As a kid, I would go with my mom to a fabric store and try to find a cloth that didn't resemble a couch or curtains—then have a seamstress piece together a dress I could wear to a wedding or a family affair. It was mortifying! But to be honest, I was happy to be covered so no one would see my body.

I have a client who used to come in, sit on my couch and put a pillow over her belly. Every time. At first, I thought it was for comfort, but then she confessed that she always finds something to place over herself so others won't see her "belly." She was hiding her "self."

She is hardly the only one to feel this way.

Before launching 2B Mindset with Beachbody, I watched hours and hours of confessions from folks who wanted to test-drive the plan, and the number one common belief—the thing every person said— was that they didn't feel like their personalities matched their bodies. I immediately related to their thinking—I remember feeling trapped in a body I didn't want—but I finally realized that the negative mindset was only holding me back. Catch yourself next time you find yourself criticizing your looks. Reshape your narrative to something more encouraging and productive. Working with me, and trusting the process, will teach you to reconnect to your body and appreciate the evolution of your shape and curves at every stage, starting with where you are now and every point leading up to where you ultimately want to be.

OLD MINDSET: *Everything Feels Hard and Will Only Get Harder*
NEW MINDSET: *Put in the Effort and It Will Become Effortless*

Not to overstate it, but this might very well be the biggest differentiating factor between the 2B Mindset and every other diet or program you've done in the past. People always seem to anticipate plateaus before they even occur. I can't tell you how often people wrongfully believe that weight loss gets harder as you get closer to your goal weight. That is simply not true.

By eating sufficient amounts of veggies, protein, FFCs and accessories throughout the day, you should be losing fat while maintaining your muscle mass and keeping up a healthy metabolism. By the time

2B MINDSET SUCCESS STORY

Michael S., 50, New York, New York, lost 38.5 pounds in 3 months*

"I feel more confident than ever!"

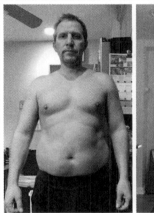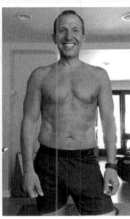

Results vary depending on starting point and effort.

SINCE FOOD IS the fuel we need to run our body, diet can have a serious impact on our energy level—both mental and physical. When Michael first heard about 2B Mindset, his poor dietary choices had him physically and mentally exhausted, leaving him with zero motivation to exercise. Additionally, his cholesterol levels were elevated, and most of his clothes were too tight. After just three months on 2B Mindset, he not only dropped over 38 pounds—but also ended up with some impressively chiseled abs. "I feel great!" he tells me. "Everything has changed and I feel more confident than ever."

His new and improved healthy diet gives his body the fuel it needs for regular workout sessions, he says, and guess what? His clothes fit once again! "I have been able to maintain a healthy weight by following the basic guidelines of 2B Mindset," he adds. "It's a pretty simple way to live once you know it."

Michael is using the lessons of my program and he encourages others to do the same. "Don't wait another second," he says. "Start at your next meal. It's very simple—just have to get that mindset!"

you are within a few pounds of your goal weight, you should have a clear idea of your weight-loss days, go-to meals, regular routine and healthy habits, so that it will feel effortless to keep it going. That's why I keep saying: "Put in the effort to become effortless."

It may feel like pushing a monster truck tire up a hill at times, but when you stay positive and stick with it, eventually that tire will roll right down the other side, which is how I describe what Melting Mode

The Power of Positive Thinking

I cringe when I hear someone use the dreaded word "fat" to describe their body. When people use this extremely negative word, it almost always leads to a negative outcome. Here's a hypothetical example: Let's say a person really believes "I'm so fat" before going to a party. Are they going to feel great getting dressed? No. Are they going to be that excited to see people? No. They're probably feeling really uncomfortable and miserable, and so by the time they get to the party, they're already feeling like crap.

Let's say the pizza comes out. They might think, *Well, I'm so fat anyway, I might as well have a slice, or three.* And then, *I already had the pizza, now I might as well have some French fries, some pretzels and heck, why not more pizza?* That's followed by, *Well, I blew off the day anyway. I'm so fat, I might as well have some cake.* Then they may leave the party, go home, run into the kitchen and eat some more—but they certainly do not want to track it all. Oh, no. And it's very likely they will not want to get on the scale the next morning, either. This can lead to a downward spiral of emotional eating that can last weeks or even months.

Let's compare that to a more positive outlook. I'll use myself as an example. I like to start a day when I'm in weight-loss mode thinking, *I'm losing weight every day, and today will be a weight loss day.* So let's say I'm feels like. You will get there.

You've conquered stuff like this before. If you start flossing after forgetting to for a while, the first couple of days, you're bleeding everywhere and it's a disgusting, painful mess, but then it becomes effortless and that's your new habit. Every September, parents freak out because getting into the swing of school is tough—your kids sleep late, you're packing their lunches again, the checklist is a mile long. But then two

---

invited to that same party. I go in thinking, *I want to make today a weight loss day!* I want to go to this party to enjoy it and talk to people. So that's really the first thing I focus on. And then, if I want to have something, it's "Water First." And if I'm feeling hungry, it's, "Veggies Most."

If I'm really in weight-loss mode, then I might have found out in advance whether or not the hosts planned to serve veggies and maybe brought a veggie platter with me—or I've made a good salad (or suggested that I could). However I go about it, I've just made sure there will be something there that I can fill up on. Sure, there may be pizza at parties, but it's a weight-loss day, so I'm going to look for leaner proteins to keep me full. And sure, they might serve cake, but I may think, *Do I need this eating opportunity? DINTEO? You know, I could save that for another time because today's a great day and I want to see great results.*

Of course, I continue to enjoy the people I'm with and I leave the party thinking, *I rock. That was really excellent.* I can't wait to track it all, and I'm actually looking forward to going on the scale the next morning to see how it all played out.

This sort of approach just keeps spiraling into increasingly positive feelings and better food choices for weeks and weeks to come. A positive mindset creates more positive actions—and a stronger sense of control and empowerment.

Ilana-ism

Make Today a Weight-Loss Day

When you choose to "make today a weight-loss day," you drop your excuses and work toward a plan of improvement. This way of thinking is what helps you bust through plateaus and keeps you progressing forward. Whether the scale went up or down this morning, within this program, there is always room for growth. Some simple changes that can lead to big results:

- Have you only been tracking once at the end of the day? How about today you track right after each meal for better recall.

- Have you been settling for your minimum water goal? How about remembering the More? Sure! model before going for seconds at dinner, which will also get you drinking more ounces.

weeks in, you think, "This is the best thing ever! My kids are in school all day!" Everyone gets it together. Change is good. Change is essential. Step up your effort, remind yourself that you can handle the challenges that come with change and eventually these positive changes will become part of your effortless routine.

OLD MINDSET: *Everyone's Judging Me*
NEW MINDSET: *I Need to Focus More on Improving the Way I Talk to and Treat Myself and Care Less about What Others May Be (but Likely Aren't) Thinking*

I know from experience: When you're overweight, you can have a constant fear that people are looking at your body and your plate. I thought about it all the time. Almost every overweight person I've ever counseled has mentioned a concern about what others might think. I've also seen this in people who just need to lose a few pounds but feel self-conscious about their bodies—they think everyone is staring, thinking the worst about the "fat slob" wedging into the rideshare or in line at the local burger joint. When I work with them and recommend that they order their own entree rather than share plates of fried apps or that they bring a new veggie-based dish, not their famous cookies, to the potluck, they push back with concern over what others might think. The sooner you choose to care more about your own opinion of yourself than the possible, but maybe even fictitious, thoughts of others, the better off you'll be.

In reality, other people are usually busy focusing on their own lives. And the more fit, confident, goal-oriented, healthy and proud you truly are, the more work you're dedicating to that focus and those results. If you were eating next to a thin, successful stranger, and then afterward, a reporter asked her what you ordered for lunch, she'd likely have no idea. She was probably more focused on her next presentation, upcoming event, her own delicious salad or answering her text. Anyone who is focused too much on others isn't focusing enough on themselves. You can drop these insecurities by catching them and changing your thinking toward your own self-care and what you can do that will make your own self proud.

OLD MINDSET: *I'm Starving!*
NEW MINDSET: *I'm Hungry and I'm Okay*

It's kind of a diet cliché to complain that you're "starving—absolutely starving!" I find that to be a very unproductive and desperate word. Just think about what it means, and how strong it is. Maybe it's because there are people who are *actually* starving, and so it hits a different chord with me, but I also work with clients who say it more often than they realize, and I see the consequences. When you say this phrase, it puts you in a vulnerable and dramatic mindset. And it's not even true.

The truth is, if you ate in the past 48 hours, you're not starving. I'll ask my clients, "Did you have breakfast this morning?" They'll say, "Yeah, but I haven't eaten in like three hours." I tell them, "Then you're hungry. Not starving."

Being hungry isn't fun but if you haven't planned ahead or become very busy, it could happen. We may get hungry, but hunger doesn't require an impulsive reaction. It's a gradual sensation and never too important to bypass logical thinking. If you're hungry, drink Water First, eat Veggies Most. No need to exaggerate. I'm guilty of doing this at times myself, but exaggerated characterizations lead to exaggerated choices that never make you feel great. I'll hear people coming off an airplane, saying they're "starving." Instead of waiting a few more steps to find a banana and yogurt at the next coffee shop, they scarf down the first thing they see, which is usually an overpriced, tasteless, cellophane-coated muffin.

There is a lot of potential when you tell yourself "I'm okay." Next time you find yourself using overblown statements like "I was terrible," "I'm obsessed with that dessert," or "I'm dying for a slice," remind yourself that you're okay and stronger than you think. Interestingly enough, we can survive about three weeks without food and about three days without water but only a little over three minutes without breath. Whenever you feel a slight sense of panic, especially as it relates to your hunger, bring your attention to breathing in and breathing out, and remind yourself that you're okay.

Oops, I Overate

Saying that you will always be in control and eat mindfully isn't realistic, even for people who mostly do. Alcohol, holiday parties, stress, large portions and highly addictive foods can get in the way and contribute to an episode of overeating. But rather than feeling like a failure, consider it a learning experience, and follow it with these steps.

- *Lose the Shame.* Like I said, it happens to everyone, even fit and highly disciplined people you wouldn't suspect. It's part of the human process.

- *Believe in Yourself.* One episode—or a period of overeating—doesn't mean that it's the end. It's never too late to pull it together; you will still be able to reach your goals.

- *Reflect.* What could you have done differently to prevent it? Made your own dinner rather than rush to order? Drank more water? Chosen a dish with more veggies and ate them first? Threw it out or put it away when you'd had enough?

- *Annihilate the Threat.* Clearly identify the foods that caused you to spiral and remove them from your space. If there are leftovers worth redeeming, wrap them up to bring to a friend. If it is just junk that wouldn't benefit anyone, then recognize it's better in the trash than in your body. Don't continue to rebuy the foods that trigger you; remove them from your path.

- *Track It and Move on.* Don't pretend it didn't happen and "start again tomorrow." You don't have to wait for later to get it together; you can bounce back stronger and reduce the chances of a repeat—if you take the time now to write it all down. Then you can focus on your 2 Bunnies and 2B Mindset plan for a better tomorrow.

SPECIAL SECTION

OLD MINDSET/NEW MINDSET FOR SILLY TREATS

ALWAYS SAY YOU can have it all, but not all at once. You can't expect to go to a party and have the chips, soda, Twizzlers, pizza *and* cake, even if you try telling yourself that you'll start again tomorrow. This is true not only if your goal is weight loss, but if you just hope to have a healthy, well-functioning body. And your kids shouldn't eat or expect to eat everything, either. Get picky with silly treats. Stick with one thing, and make it your favorite thing.

This really worked for me. I was stuck for a while at around 185 pounds, annoyed that I couldn't lose more. One day, I overheard someone say, "If it's not chocolate, it's not worth it." I gave this philosophy a try and *BAM!*—I slid right down to the 150s. I was wasting so much time with pumpkin pie and berry tarts. It didn't matter if I asked for "just a sliver," or scooped out the filling and left the buttery crust untouched. It turns out that they were never worth it for me. Once I started politely passing up non-chocolate treats, I started feeling so much better and didn't feel like I had to sacrifice much to do so. (I got very lucky and married the yin to my yang on this one, because

Ilana-ism

Better in the Waste Than on Your Waist

Don't suck up your kids' last bites of sandwich or leftover pieces of scrambled egg because they were intuitive enough to leave them there. You don't need to be the hero who brings home the leftover cakes and chocolates. You're not a vacuum cleaner, and it's better in the waste than on your waist.

those are Noah's favorite desserts. That was a real dealmaker! Since his favorite sweet treats, like peach cobbler and apple strudel, don't tempt me, it makes it easier for me to stay on track when he has them.)

Over time, I would experiment with cheesecake, pecan pie and Snickerdoodles, but as I got thinner and happier on the 2B Mindset—with tracking especially—I really eased them out. My one exception to the rule is ice cream, because chocolate ice cream isn't always the best flavor, and I freaking love ice cream. (As did my mom and as does my daughter, which makes me wonder if these preferences are nature or nurture.)

Think about your favorite sweets. What are they? List them out, in order of preference, here:

_____

_____

_____

_____

_____

_____

Whatever you pick, own it. You can love and enjoy these things, even become a connoisseur of the category! In fact, becoming a bit of a snob about your favorite item is a must. It makes you appreciate it so much more. Noah is a gummy guy. (Again, bless his soul, because gummies don't interest me. I'd rather chew fruit-flavored gum). His big caveat is that they need to be "soft and fresh." When we go to the movies, he will feel around the bags for the "freshest" feeling ones so he can maximize his enjoyment. He doesn't care if he looks a bit goofy because it makes for a completely elevated experience. And if they don't feel right, he won't waste his time (or his money). This is how it should be. This is how the French stay so slim while enjoying sweets. They are "mindful" about their indulgences and choosy when it comes to quality, ambiance and ingredients.

I know that sounds like a fantasy, but that's my job, to show you how that "naturally skinny" way of thinking is actually attainable when you let me help you change your mindset and behaviors.

Part of "owning" your silly treats is also recognizing them for what they are. Here, I've included some New Mindset definitions. They may sound brutally honest, but remember, I've had to be brutally honest with myself in order to help me get to this point. You don't have to agree with any of them to be successful, and if any of these are your "one thing" that's okay too, but my clients love to hear this blunt, refreshing and underrepresented viewpoint, so I think it's better that you hear it, too.

- ■ ***Pancakes* = *cake!*** *There is no difference.* And no, you can't taste any of that hidden cream and buttermilk after you've plunged them under syrup. You want pancakes and syrup? Make the 2B Mindset banana egg pancakes or a high-protein pancake mix—you really can't tell the difference. Pancakes are also never worth it as breakfast on a vacation when you know you'll probably want something great like actual cake or a cocktail later on in the day.

- ■ ***Doughnuts* = *deep fried dough.*** I have a friend who is "naturally thin" and loves doughnuts. (I know. Annoying, right?) But then again, this person makes a point to only savor doughnuts—not all things with dough. She's very picky about how fresh, hot and amazing a doughnut has to be to be worth it and can give you a detailed review of the best and worst in town. So although doughnuts are "her favorite thing," she is prewired with the Push Off Method, so she only eats three or four a year. By the way, if the filling is your thing (custard, chocolate, jam, etc.), you can pull apart the doughnut and enjoy the insides. Just dollop it on a plate, and using a fork or strawberry, eat, savor and enjoy. You should never feel forced to eat more than you want because that is a form of wasting food, too.

- ***Chocolate* = *not always chocolate*.** Real chocolate is made from cocoa, which resembles ground coffee—it's bitter, low sugar and very high in fiber. The chocolate candy we see around Valentine's Day has very little actual chocolate in it. Choose dark chocolate, or better yet, choose chocolate brands that list a percentage on the label and aim for at least 50 percent real chocolate. (I prefer 75 percent and above.) The realer the chocolate, the more it hits the chocolate fix. Nowadays, it's my main focus when it comes to sweets. I'll even pick the chips out of a chocolate chip cookie to get the best (and only the best) part for me. And here's a dirty secret for you: White chocolate doesn't even have any chocolate in it! When I learned this, I had to stop including it in my preferred chocolate list (and I dropped another five pounds).

- ***Cake* = *sugary, fatty bread*.** Any baking show clearly shows you that to make cake, you start with white flour and egg, followed by a tornado of oil, butter and sugar. To minimize temptation, select a single favorite flavor, style or type. My father-in-law is a genius at this because his favorite cake is carrot cake, and how often are you faced with that? He usually has it no more than once a year, on his birthday, when everyone makes it for him. And don't choose "birthday cake" as your favorite, especially if you spend time with family. There is always a birthday. Therefore, there's always a birthday cake. If you want it that bad, I recommend having a good birthday cake backup, like the Birthday Cake Shakeology (see recipe on page 176).

  Another trick is to be more choosy about specifying a unique bakery that makes an incredible special-order birthday cake that you don't want to live without. Skip grocery store cakes and box mixes—not because they aren't delicious, but because they are too ordinary and you can enjoy them at any time, so you definitely don't need them now in weight loss mode.

- ***Pasta* = *bowl of paste*.** Chances are you don't *love* plain pasta. What you probably really enjoy is the flavor-packed sauce or gobs of salted butter that it's tossed in. Here's a way to still enjoy it: What sauce do you miss? You want the fancy restaurant's penne alla vodka sauce? You can ask for it in a side bowl with a spoon or with a side order of steamed vegetables so you can create your own fantasy dish that's Veggies Most. Or ask for some to go and put it on top of zoodles at home! You'll still get the yummy flavor you love. It does the trick, I promise. If you really want to try a pasta dish, continue to order a Plate It dinner and ask to share some with someone else at the table. View it as a silly carb treat within the More? Sure! model so you can get back to your roasted artichokes if you find yourself yearning for more.

■ **Rice = *just a vehicle*.** Unless it's crispy like tadig (a Persian delicacy), rice is usually not doing much more than mopping up your curry sauce or holding together your sushi. White rice is also nutritionally pointless, filled with refined carbs and lacking fiber. Don't waste your time unless you're in Japan and it feels like *Jiro Dreams of Sushi*. And if you love a side of rice and beans with your Mexican takeout order, ask them to hold the rice and simply cook up some cauliflower rice with a sprinkle of taco seasoning. It's just as tasty and definitely more satisfying.

■ **One Sushi Roll = *about three slices of white bread*.** Is this reality a total buzzkill or what? It's pretty shocking that a standard California roll contains the carb exchange of 2½ to 4 slices of bread. And a spicy tuna roll is not much different than a heavy mayo tuna sandwich, similar to what you'd get from a 7-Eleven. As a treat, these 600–700 calorie rolls aren't so bad, but the lack of protein, fiber and veggies won't likely keep you full. Instead, focus on eating protein and veggies like edamame, a cucumber or green salad, and some sashimi or cooked fish. Then order a hand roll or two that are either light on brown rice or wrapped in cucumber or just seaweed and rice-less. For more tips for what to order in restaurants, like Japanese and Thai, refer to the 2B Mindset video.

■ **French Fries / Fish Sticks / Chicken Nuggets = *all taste the same*.** Think about it. You may think you love one or all of them, but none have that distinct a flavor, especially when dunked in ketchup. Remember, foods are most addictive when they possess a mix of sugar (ketchup), salt and fat (fried anything). So only start—aka at the end of the More? Sure! model—if you have a plan to stop.

- *Egg Nog* = *heavy cream.*

- *Beer* = *liquid bread.*

- *Movie Theatre Popcorn* = *like chowing down on a stick of melted butter or drinking salted oil.*

OLD MINDSET: *I Shouldn't Be Eating This*

NEW MINDSET: *I'm Fully Enjoying This*

Eating and thinking are connected. And I have a phrase that really helps me, which is "I'm fully enjoying this." When I go in for a piece of chocolate mousse, or when I go in for some popcorn, or when I go in for, say, a fried tempura, piece of sushi or a slice of white mushroom pizza, I like to say, "I'm going to fully enjoy this." And while I am eating it, I actually like to think, *I'm fully enjoying this, I'm fully enjoying this.* And if you're not, then just drop the fork. It's not worth having it if you're not enjoying it.

Ilana-ism

Treat, Not Cheat!

If you're having a yummy treat, make sure that you actually enjoy it! Too many times people feel guilty about eating decadent food, but it's time to make over that mindset because what is the point of having it if you are not even enjoying it? See more about this on page 252.

OLD MINDSET: *I Hate the Scale, I'm Scared of What it Says*

NEW MINDSET: *The Scale is My Friend, It Helps Me Be More Self-Aware*

You learned why the scale is a fundamental part of 2B Mindset in Chapter 2. But as I wrote in the *Nutrition & Food Science Interna-*

tional Journal, I feel as though people overthink going on the scale and correlate it with a powerful emotional experience when it really just has to serve as a quick health check-in. I know you may still "hate" the scale, because you either associate it with a bad diet or have avoided it for a long time, but just know that you can learn to love it in the future.

After having my son Julian, I was 21 pounds heavier postpartum. I couldn't and wouldn't have been able to lose that weight without having a positive and sensible relationship with the scale. It didn't define me when I weighed 215 pounds, and it doesn't define me now. It isn't bad or mean when it goes up, but it does help me constantly learn how to develop a better relationship with food and myself, especially because each stage of life can require different eating techniques. For instance, after my mother passed away, people convinced me to eat chocolate to make me feel better. Unfortunately, I fell for it temporarily and ate a bunch of things I didn't even take pleasure in. Thankfully, even though my head was a mess and I was not thinking clearly, the scale opened my eyes and helped me stop it.

It helped me see that I needed emotional healing, not emotional eating. It helped me find myself again at a time when I could have totally let myself and health go, which wouldn't be anything my mother would have wanted. Without the scale helping me approach my efforts in an objective and logical way, I would never have been able to get to, and maintain, where I am today—both physically and mentally.

OLD MINDSET: *Should I Be "Bad" or "Good"?*
NEW MINDSET: *I Could Feel Sluggish and Regretful or Ensure That I Feel Energized and Proud*

My biggest pet peeve is when a private client calls herself "bad" for eating certain foods. We need to let go of judgment and approach food and ourselves with a greater sensibility and a more positive mindset. You're

Ilana-ism

JOMO, aka "Joy of Missing Out," aka the opposite of FOMO, fear of missing out.

Every time you say no to something, you say yes to something else.
A pass on late-night munchies is a wake-up to a weight loss.
A pass on a cocktail can mean a deeper night's sleep. Every choice
comes with sacrifice, and the healthier choice is not one you will regret.

never bad if you have a brownie, but you have to be honest with yourself and ask if you're feeling proud of that choice and going to enjoy it. So many people tell me that as they're eating, they feel guilty and that is just sad. You need to be honest with yourself and see that your state of negativity and "being bad" is likely perpetuating those actions. You have the capacity to change at any point and begin to act in the way you want to.

OLD MINDSET: *Taking Care of My Health Is an Expense*
NEW MINDSET: *Taking Care of My Health Is an Investment*

To find reasons why losing this weight will save you money or make you money, I worked with a nursing home owner and developer who lost 40 pounds, watched his business soar and has kept it off throughout its growth. Even when catching up with him currently in Maintenance Mode, he told me that when he's five pounds leaner, he swears he feels sharper. Excess weight—or a preoccupation with food—can distract you and weigh down your energy. It can hinder your confidence or cause you to spend more on even bigger clothes—a big expense to pay financially and emotionally.

Take stock of how this might apply to you. I'm not trying to be superficial here—if you're a brilliant real estate agent, your knowledge and experience will help you sell homes regardless. But how will you sell homes differently, how would it affect your presentations and showings, if you felt leaner, trimmer and swifter?

Also, when you track and learn your best weight-loss meals, you can streamline your eating plan. It makes it quicker and cheaper to shop and buy in bulk and makes you less reliant on restaurant meals and more dependent on leaner DIY meals that leave you with leftovers to take with you the next day. You shouldn't ever feel that losing weight with the 2B Mindset requires a ton of money. If anything, people save a lot of money because, as you might notice from the 4-Week Slim-Down Plan, each day of food can be made for less than what you probably spent the last time you went to a restaurant.

OLD MINDSET: *I Work Out for My Physical Health*
NEW MINDSET: *I Work Out for My Mental Health*

What's one word to describe how you feel after a workout? I can't pick just one. It's Confident, Secure, Focused, Centered, Energetic, Grateful, Motivated and so much more. Yes, there are physical benefits of exercise. It lowers blood sugar and blood pressure, and can help prevent bone fractures and arthritis. These are all helpful for your long-term health. Yet the mental health benefits of relieving anxiety, stress, insecurity and lethargy are also important. When you exercise you are kinder and more positive to those around you. It's seriously the greatest gift we can give to ourselves and those we love. Our emotions are in overdrive, especially around changing seasons and major life events! One way to ease your mind and silence self-doubt is a workout. I never underestimate its benefits for boosting my mood.

2B MINDSET **SUCCESS STORY**

Deanna P., 50, Weehawken, New Jersey, lost 18.5 pounds in 3.5 months*

"Fifty is the new twenty-five!"

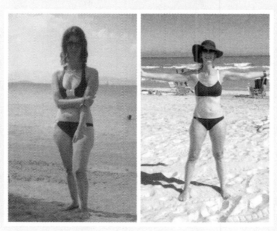

*Results vary depending on starting point and effort

HAVE SEEN 2B MINDSET basically put years back on a person's life or helped them look years younger, and Deana is a great example. She was about to turn 50, and was 20 pounds heavier than she had been just three years prior when she got married. "I felt fat, bloated, depressed and hopeless!" she says, explaining that she would lose a few pounds, just to gain it back again. "It was awful being stuck in that cycle."

She was determined to look and feel her very best when she turned 50, so she gave the program a shot—and it proved to be one of the best decisions of her life. Using the principles of the program, she drank lots of water, consumed a plethora of veggies, ate healthier foods overall, plated her meals, weighed herself daily and started journaling—and hasn't stopped since.

"I am in awe of the fact that I could get this thin," she exclaims after losing over 18 pounds. "I am not pear-shaped anymore. It's truly amazing!" With her new figure has come a sense of confidence. "Fifty is the new twenty-five! It's true what they say: knowledge is power. I feel like I can do anything. I know if I put my mind to something, all things are possible!"

CHAPTER SUMMARY

If you change your mindset, your choices can come from empowerment and enjoyment, not deprivation and despair. Some of my favorite new ways of thinking include:

■ OLD MINDSET: *I Will Never Lose All This Weight*

NEW MINDSET: *I Can Do Anything, Focus on Two Pounds at a Time*

■ OLD MINDSET: *I Gained Weight and I Feel Gross*

NEW MINDSET: *It's Okay, I Can Drop It*

■ OLD MINDSET: *I Have to Eat Healthier*

NEW MINDSET: *I Get to Eat Healthier*

■ OLD MINDSET: *Everything Is Hard Before It Gets Better*

NEW MINDSET: *Put in the Effort to Become Effortless*

■ OLD MINDSET: *Everyone's Judging Me*

NEW MINDSET: *I Need to Focus More on Myself*

■ OLD MINDSET: *I Hate the Scale, I'm Scared of What It Says*

NEW MINDSET: *The Scale Is My Friend, It Helps Me Be More Self-Aware*

■ OLD MINDSET: *I Work Out for My Physical Health*

NEW MINDSET: *I Work Out for My Mental Health*

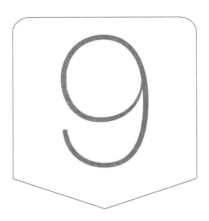

STOP THE SELF-SABOTAGE

Excuses Are Not Your Friend.
So Quit Making Them.

YOU'RE TIRED OF treating your body like a garbage can. You want to not feel disgusting anymore, and to never feel disgusting again. What will it take for you to stop making excuses so you can get out of your own way?

Start by finding your excuses in this chapter, and we can cross them off together.

Why do we self-sabotage? I think people self-sabotage when they are frustrated: they feel like they're eating well and they're not losing weight. Frustration brings on self-sabotage. So does believing you're not worth it—but you *are* worth it. You're always worth it.

I've definitely sabotaged myself in the past. I think everyone does. For me, it took a while, but after years of being obese, I realized I had energy and positivity to share with the world, but my exterior wasn't matching the way I really felt—or the way I wanted to live. I became fed up with making excuses and accepted the fact that I could take control of it instead. When my size 20 jeans were becoming snug and I knew size 22 would mean I couldn't even fit into Gap and Old Navy's extended sizes, it hit me that I would be forced to shop in plus-size-only stores. This was particularly difficult to accept given that my friends at the time were still shopping in the juniors' section.

So I stopped and dropped the self-sabotage.

The key to stopping self-sabotage is understanding the push and pull between discipline and surrender. One aspect of being human, I've discovered by working with thousands of people in private practice and at UCLA, is that we all crave discipline. A lot of clients come to me with, "I'm so over it." They're at their absolute highest weight, and they've overindulged beyond belief. "I just want to be disciplined," they say. "Just tell me what to eat."

But we also all crave surrender. A perfect illustration of this is what happens every January first when people say, "I'm going to do this crazy diet! I'm going to do keto. I'm going to do a fast. I'm going to cut out this. I'm going to cut out that. I'm going to cut out *everything* and I'm going to lose weight." Then they exercise that sense of discipline—until that human side of them comes in, and they surrender to chips and mini hot dogs.

It's easy to see why. If you've been a food-focused, food-obsessed stress eater—and love the taste of really good food—it's going to take some work. Believe me, I can relate. These have been identities we've created and reinforced with eating patterns for months or even years. I can't snap my fingers and expect to lose that whole aspect of me that loves to indulge, and you won't either. It takes about a one-year cycle of practice, getting through all the different holidays, stressors and celebrations to feel truly confident in your changed gravitation. To this day, when I get really stressed, or when I feel like I want to indulge, that craving doesn't go away. But I've gotten better with practice, with time, with the Ilana-isms, with viewing this all as a process and with 2B Mindset. You're always either losing weight or learning from it. There is no room for self-sabotage, only self-strength. I've gotten stronger and stronger and stronger. *You* will get stronger and stronger and stronger, too. But for right now, know yourself, don't test yourself. Don't start with the fries if you know you usually clear the fries. Keep yourself in a disciplined state with food because it feels great when you do.

EVERY SUCCESSFUL COMPETITOR HAS A COMPETITIVE EDGE. THIS IS YOURS.

T HE STRUGGLE BETWEEN the real you and the self-sabotaging you is a true battle. And it's important to fight it so you can defeat negative self-talk and old habits. Every successful competitive athlete relies on a routine, set of rituals, favorite gear, lucky spots and specific schedule requirements. They don't feel bad about these quirks; they lean into them. People have so many tips and tools that feed into continuous self-sabotage—like rebuying those chocolates, turning to your cozy pants and kicking the scale to the curb. But once you find a tool, tip or behavior that *assists* in your weight loss and wellness plan, I need you to lean into it now.

Don't get in your way and tell yourself you shouldn't need to buy that yummy vinaigrette because you can make your own if you know you'll eat much more salad and lose more weight. Buy the dressing. Better yet, if it's shelf stable, buy a few at a time. You may even want to keep one at a family member's house or your office, or gift one to a friend who wants to eat better too. Don't apologize for needing tools—every successful person has them, so put yourself in the group.

Some worthwhile tools and investments that can help defeat self-sabotage are:

- *A comfortable pair of athletic shoes that encourage you to take walks*

- *A Shakeology subscription to satisfy your sweet cravings on a daily basis in a way that fuels your body best*

- *Sunday trips to the farmers' market, which can be slightly more expensive but get you more excited for your veggie-packed week ahead*

- *A fancy new knife set to make chopping a breeze*

- *New spins on dessert like teas, sparkling waters, marinades or seasoning blends to add enjoyment to your dishes/meals*

Arm yourself with solutions that help you foster healthy habits and silence the self-sabotage. Mental and physical health are wealth. You need to value and prioritize what makes you feel your best.

My clients and I talk about this all the time. I've collected their most common excuses, and I thought I'd share my advice with you here. Find the excuses that resonate most with you, and let's tackle them together, once and for all.

"I hate my body but can't change it."

You can change your body. Start by changing the way you *think* about your body. Start by looking at your body part of concern, like your back, stomach or knees, the same way that you look at your children, or animals you love or whatever is most precious to you. Nurture them. Your mind's wants are not more important than your body's needs. I had a client who thought working out midday was too indulgent, because she thought she should be doing something productive instead. I told her, "When you exercise, it might seem 'indulgent,' but it makes your back better. Would you not take your kids to the dentist because it seems indulgent? You have to do it. Your body needs and wants to move, so set it in the calendar, alert your family that you'll be away if you need to and get going!"

The same goes with eating. You feel like you want the side of fries, you think you deserve them because you didn't get them last night. Override your propensity to get in your own way. This issue could stem from a fear of succeeding or something even deeper that you may want to work out in therapy, but in the meantime, don't let it cause your body to suffer. Confront that challenging inner voice and choose the side salad instead. Once you're finished, you'll be glad you did. You know you can do it again because you've now done it once before. Feel proud of yourself for demonstrating a smart choice.

"I love junk food."

Welcome to the human race. Wanting to just binge one night—to eat chocolate chip cookies, gummy bears and pizza in your pajamas— that's something we would all want to do, every one of us. The issue is that it comes with consequences that we know we can't sustain. We know those nights cause us to feel bloated, lazy, heavy, and send us down a vicious cycle of wanting to repeat it. But the initial craving is not necessarily the problem. The area that we want to work on is: Why are we having this craving? What is making us feel so wound up that we're so desperate to let go? What's another way to express that sense of liberation and freedom to "do whatever we want" that we won't regret? What's a more kosher vice? How much do we have to release to feel complete? Are there better ways of doing it? So that instead of saying: "I need to cut everything out" or "I need to just binge and binge and binge" and then Friday night leads to Saturday leads to Sunday leads to, "I'll start Monday" leads to Wednesday, or leads to next month....

5 Ways to Steel Yourself Against Self-Sabotage

■ *1. Pull Out the Calendar.* Setting timely goals is one of the most effective ways my clients stay consistent. People like to make broad goals like "I want to lose 10 pounds," but it's not good enough. *Set a date.* When you are faced with chocolate cookies at four p.m, or nine p.m., it's too easy to say, "Ehh, it's okay, I can have some." However, if you know that you want to lose 10 pounds by that big presentation you're giving or an event you are attending, things will change. It will help you stay more focused and able to say, "Nah, I really don't need cookies right now" and instead look up a picture of the event space and start to visualize yourself there at your goal.

■ *2. Make a Realistic Plan.* I am obsessed with making people feel full and in control in eating situations so that they can stay consistent. If they feel too hungry and overwhelmed, most people will "fall off" and lose their stride. Just because your meeting went late, you didn't sleep enough and you didn't get to meal prep, that doesn't mean you should eat a bunch of tacos and nachos for dinner. You need to know that you can still order takeout, eat at a buffet or even raid your freezer and still eat well. Life is never consistent, so you need an unconditional plan that works with your life—like the Enjoy Takeout Food video in 2B Mindset, where I walk you through a stack of menus and what you can order from every cuisine to stay on track.

■ *3. Play Out the Plan.* Sometimes I hear a client get a little too confident about her ability to control an eating situation, and I'll make her go deeper into ironing out the details. It's very easy to say, "I'm going to that party, but don't worry, I won't be tempted by anything. I'll be fine." While I love the confidence and enthusiasm, I know (from working with hundreds of very smart and successful people) that more planning is needed to build true self-control. We may think we have the big idea until we start sipping champagne within snacking range of the sushi bar and chocolate fountain—or even the sad, store-bought cookie, pretzel and mini-donut table. That is why I help my clients walk through the event so that, when they see the pass-around appetizers (or whatever else tempts them), they can clearly visualize themselves going to the bar to get Water First and keep their two hands on the wheel so they can use the Push Off Method until they find some veggie-based options.

■ *4. Learn to Politely Pass.* We are faced with more than 200 eating decisions every day. Thousands if you're going grocery food shopping or ordering from delivery apps with dozens of online menus to choose from. We pass vending machines and snacks everywhere we go, and then there are all of the sweets and treats our friends, family and coworkers offer us. It's endless and can really hinder our ability to stay focused. It's important to use DINTEO—remember, it stands for "Do I Need This Eating Opportunity?"—to help you stay mindful.

When you do pass, rather than saying, "No," use my mom's great line, "No thanks, I'm good." I love this phrase because "No thanks" is quick and polite and "I'm good" is a friendly reminder that you *are* good and gives you a sense of empowerment.

■ *5. Find Accountability.* Accountability is great because, in those moments of weakness, you'll want a reminder to stay on track. Accountability can come in many forms. For instance, if you're in the habit of tracking your food, you may not have a second helping if you know you have to write it down. It's a great idea to seek someone to help as well. My clients and family love the added sense of accountability I provide. You can become a certified 2B Mindset mentor, in which I share my best tips for coaching people through this program, and that can help you coach yourself through it, too.

what can you do? What can you do before you surrender so much that you've gone to extremes?

The solution is to find more productive, less destructive vices and points of surrender.

For example, I work with a lot of moms and, as a busy mom myself, I understand that your mind is thinking about a zillion things all the time. So after the kids go to sleep, you just want to give in to the candy, junk food, wine, chips—to the entire pantry, essentially! And that's the habit.

Instead: Ditch the kitchen and go straight to the bedroom with a sparkling water or yummy tea and Pinterest kitchen ideas or DIY projects for the next hour. Sleep in one day. Book a massage using Groupon. Plan a concert, karaoke, museum or comedy club date with friends. Sneak a quick TV show in the middle of an afternoon, maybe a childhood favorite. Reserve the breast-feeding room at work and meditate or stretch. Shop online for some soon-to-fit goal pants (choose ones you can easily return if they don't work out). Spend more time doing your makeup or give your skin a break and ditch the makeup altogether. Shop YouTube for organizing or skin care tips. Institute "unplugged" Friday nights at home where the whole family turns off their cell phones for game night. For me, sometimes during a workout, when it says, "This is the modifier," sometimes I go into child's pose or do the modifier and give myself credit for showing up. Other times I push myself because sweating is one of the most effective methods for releasing frustration and built-up negative energy. And when I'm really stressed, sometimes I'll do pigeon pose, which makes me feel so calm and grounded and is the utmost release.

"I'm just going to cheat anyway."

When I talk to my private clients, some will always say they "cheated" or missed steps. I always respond, "You're only cheating yourself if

2B MINDSET **SUCCESS STORY**

*Saudi A., an Independent Team Beachbody Coach, 40, New York, New York,
lost 31 pounds in 5 months**

"I knew I had to stop making excuses!"

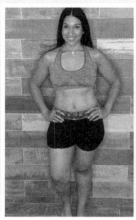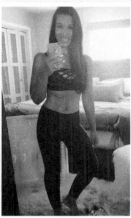

*Results vary depending on starting point and effort.

FOR MOST OF her life, Saudi attributed her voluptuous body to her genetics. She was a "curvaceous Latina," after all. However, after hearing my story she realized that she didn't have to be a slave to her genetics, and she decided to stop making excuses!

She dropped more than 30 pounds in just three months on the 2B Mindset—and hasn't gained it back. "I loved this journey, and my results," she gushes. "I completely trusted the process because I knew that I deserve to be the happiest and healthiest version of myself."

Because of the program, she makes better decisions and understands how her body responds to certain foods. She also attributes her weight loss success to her new and improved mental attitude. "I am so much happier," she says. "I learned to change the things in my life that have made me gain weight in the past."

"I love the smaller girl in the mirror, my confidence is through the roof, and it's spilling into my fitness routine and family. I have more clarity of thought, and I am a better example to others."

you're not enjoying it." Or, to put it a snappier way: Treat yourself, don't cheat yourself. If you find yourself eating and enjoying it, okay, enjoy it. If you find yourself eating and hating that you're doing it, stop. If you can't stop, try to examine why and track it in your journal.

With tracking, and following the 2B Mindset principles, you'll see that it's all a process. At certain moments of your life—like the holidays, vacation and in the summer, for example—it's possible that you have a day or weekend that you gain weight, that you're going to overindulge, that you're going to let loose a bit. I'm included in this also. A lot of people think I eat perfectly all day, but I really don't. I love cocktails and ice cream and know that really good chocolate is always worth it. But the 2B Mindset will keep you grounded and on the right path, even if you've deviated slightly from the track. The goal is to make these moments less frequent and plan ahead for them so your indulgent steak dinner may include some extra dessert and lemme-have-a-tastes—but you made sure to have Water First before the glass of wine and got clever and ordered a side of creamed spinach to mix with a side of steamed spinach so you were still Veggies Most.

With time, you'll gain a more level-headed view of your relationship with food, allowing yourself to ease up when you want but tighten the reins and refocus when you need to. You'll get a little bit more excited about being disciplined—not too disciplined, but disciplined enough to follow the principles and reap the benefits of seeing those pounds melt back off. You'll discover that the 2B Mindset, when practiced consistently, really helps you get to the point where you have a more logical and purposeful relationship with food you really enjoy. The stronger you get emotionally, the better you'll become at treating yourself not cheating yourself.

How to Reframe Negative Self-Talk

The glass half full/half empty analogy perfectly demonstrates our ability to choose what we want to see. Two people can see the same number on the scale two days in a row. One person will be thankful he didn't gain, and the other will be frustrated he didn't lose. It's all a matter of perception, and we must use our mind as a tool to work for us, not against us. Instead of focusing on the fear of failing and negative habits, try to get curious about the best possible outcome of succeeding. Sometimes it's a matter of saying it before you even believe it. For example:

IF YOU'RE THINKING:	TRY CHANGING TO:
▓ I feel disgusting and will never lose all this weight.	I will drop this weight and I will drop my doubt. I know I can lose those next two pounds. I need to get serious and stay focused. I can do it. What's my plan for the rest of the day and tomorrow?
▓ I'm such a failure, I can't believe I ate all of that.	Those foods weren't even good or worth it and made me feel terrible afterward. Next time I see them, I won't be tempted by them because I really never need to have them again, or at least not for a very long time.
▓ I want to eat, I am so stressed.	I'm too stressed and distracted to eat. I need to take a walk, call a friend or make a list of what's bothering me and figure out a solution.
▓ I gained weight, I'm so bad.	I can always lose the weight as fast as I can gain the weight. I am more focused now and excited to lose more weight this week.

SPECIAL SECTION

TREAT, NOT CHEAT!

AS YOU'VE LEARNED, I designed the Core Four principles of the 2B Mindset so you never feel deprived. After all, there's no "off limits" category. You just have to manage eating the silly foods with some smarts.

You need to treat yourself without ever cheating yourself.

Let's say you love pizza. To lose weight, you need an alternative plan for your Friday wine and pizza nights (that turn into Saturday morning cold pizza breakfasts). And you do. For a couple of weeks or a month. And you manage okay. But at some point, you get the urge to bulldoze through a whole pie yourself, and that leaves you feeling stuffed, guilty and wanting to throw in the towel on this whole weight-loss thing.

That's a classic cycle of people who yo-yo. Deprive, gorge, deprive, gorge. Lose, gain, lose, gain.

If you want to succeed at losing weight, you have to learn to treat, not cheat. "Treat, Not Cheat" ties into the power of positive vocabulary because the word "cheat" is so negative. Has anything positive ever been associated with the phrase "I cheated"? I cheated on a test. I cheated on my taxes. I cheated on a partner. It's horrible. It always leads to guilt, shame and bad outcomes. It's destructive thinking that starts the downward spiral into self-sabotage.

I have never heard someone say, "I cheated by eating a cookie, but it was so delicious and satisfying. I was so fulfilled by it! I only needed one." No, instead, I typically hear: "I cheated by eating a cookie, so then I just figured I might as well have the whole sleeve of cookies—and then I went completely off the rails, raiding the fridge and pantry. I was so bad."

I want to help you understand how you can treat yourself to delicious things without this guilt and shame. Here's how!

- **Define the meaning of the word.** First, let's define the word "treat." A treat is something that we don't necessarily need for the nourishment of our bodies. Don't say you ate the chocolate bars because you were hungry. Chocolate doesn't fulfill physical hunger. If anything, it opens up your appetite and makes you want more. You want to have it for your pleasure and to enhance your enjoyment. This includes those sillier things like pizza, white pasta. cookies, cake, cocktails or a glass of wine. We don't need them for our health, but we think it would enhance our moment, and that's okay.

- **Feel actively positive (this is worth repeating).** While you're having this treat think to yourself, *I'm fully enjoying this. I'm fully experiencing this.* I want you to never regret anything that truly made you smile. However, if it gets at all negative inside your headspace, if you start to think, *Oh God, I'm so guilty! I can't believe I'm eating this!* or, *I definitely don't want to track this!* then drop the fork. Walk away, because you're not enjoying it. Do something productive instead, like drinking water or brushing your teeth. Wait until you're further along in your weight loss and you find something that's more worth it.

- **Track your treats properly.** Write down exactly what treats you've consumed—and how many of them. You may find yourself consuming less as a result. Often, a person who thinks they're cheating will write down "cookies," "cake" or "junk" instead of something more specific, like "five cookies." And that's if they're using the tracker at all and not avoiding it in shame. When they do that, they may also avoid the scale and fall into thinking, *Whatever. I've ruined everything. I'll just start again on Monday.* So destructive! Logging the specific number of snacks you've had will help you better understand the relationship between what you're eating and the number on the scale. It's information that we can learn from.

- **Don't act shocked.** If you're going to a birthday party, office event or family function, expect food and plan for it. I work with someone who told me, "I went to my grandma's house and I couldn't resist her oat-meal cookies. They're the best."

So I said, "Okay, great. How often do you go to grandma's house?" She responded, "Every weekend."

Grandma makes cookies every time and yet, somehow, my client still acts surprised when the cookies come out. Instead, you could think, Do I really need this eating opportunity again? Could I push it off to next time and look forward to it? That delayed sense of gratifi-cation is hard at first but will feel so good while you're seeing progress toward your health goals.

- **Know yourself, don't test yourself.** Sometimes, one little bite is not fine, because it can easily spiral into a series of habits and a loss of control. It's not that one bite is "bad," but be cautious of how addic-tive these foods and habits can become. Know what foods you can't stop eating after you've started so you can manage your portions of your treats. Be real with yourself so you don't fall into "Innocent" Eating, see page 39.

- **Determine which treats were worth it.** List the treats you had and write, "This one was my absolute favorite." Then rank your second favorite. And your third favorite. Then think about why you ate your fourth favorite. How'd you really feel about those gummy bears? My clients usually write, "I just ate them because they were there." Could you have done without them? This worked for my own personal weight loss: trying to think about what made me feel super-satisfied and what was not worth it. It helps wipe away the temptation the next time you see it because, yes, there is always a next time.

- **Indulge in other "treats."** Not all treats are food. Seeing two pounds less on the scale can be an enormous treat—satisfying and gratifying. That feeling you get after an amazing workout or a yoga class, when you feel like bliss, is a treat. So is fitting into a smaller size, or hav-ing something that didn't fit before zip up just right. As mentioned before, other treats include getting a pedicure or massage, going for a hike on the weekend, playing or learning an instrument, finishing an excellent book, saving up for a trip, organizing, or working on a craft or a hobby.

■ ***Distract yourself.*** Get out of the line of fire when it comes to temptation. At a party, hold water in one hand and a plate of veggies in the other. Or keep your hands on your bag or in your pockets. Talk to people and put your back to the food so you can focus on conversations, not fighting temptations. If the dessert table is calling you, it could be a sign of physical hunger on top of your environmental hunger cues. Think about the More? Sure! model and Plate It, and spot something smart you want from the buffet like a mixed salad or grilled fish or chicken breast. It could be you are distracted by real, actual hunger and therefore want to be intentional with your choices.

■ ***If it's not hunger—just the environment and situation—distract yourself elsewhere.*** When you engage your mind in other activities, you won't focus on the food, whenever or wherever you may be.

- Jump on the computer or play video games to put your hands on a keyboard or controller. Play a challenging game like Sudoku or a crossword that gets your mind deep in thought about something completely different.

- Call a friend and get some social support—you don't even have to talk about food; just let the cravings pass as you talk about your weekend.

- Walk outside—fresh air and scenery can instantly change your current state of mind and point of focus.

- Take a nice, warm bath or shower.

- Clean out a drawer in your desk or closet.

- Head to the gym or do a quick workout right at home with Beachbody On Demand.

Sometimes, you have to be brave enough to pass on things that you used to have because you're creating a new self-narrative where you are more fit, healthy and lean every day, fit comfortably into your jeans, get positive results from the doctor, feel excited to connect with people and get out of the house, and enjoy having your picture taken. These are the *real* treats on 2B Mindset—having better health, a clearer mind and more positive energy.

6 Practical Ways
to Eat Your Treats Responsibly

- *Make Treats Less Silly.* Some silly treats can become less silly and still bring you enjoyment. For instance, if you want juice, water it down. Ask for just a sliver of cake. If you love to drink tequila with sugary juices or sodas, it may be just as fun to have the tequila mixed with seltzer water and lime. Or if you're baking, sometimes you can replace oil with unsweetened applesauce in a recipe; it doesn't change the taste but seriously lowers the fat. In fact, it can make it moister and slightly sweeter. You get the same pleasure and will still track and treat it like a treat, but it's definitely a little less silly, and better for other people you may be sharing it with as well.

- *Choose High-Protein Options.* Low-protein sweets make you hungrier and wanting more later. High-protein sweets satisfy you so you eat less later. Protein shakes, like the Shakeology recipes in this book, and protein bars or light ice creams can make for some decent choices here.

- *Stick to Single-Serving Sizes.* One square of deliciously good quality chocolate can be more satisfying than a whole bar. I like to take that one square and dip it into a vanilla chamomile tea so it gets a little melty. That way the tea fills me up, and I still get my chocolate fix. It's an enhanced experience—and easier to track. Or enjoy one cookie, one cupcake or one glass of wine—and track it simply. You can see the end point, as opposed to handfuls of nuts and chips or a bag of gummy worms.

■ ***Taste like the French Do.*** If you are having something silly and the serving is large and open ended, you never have to finish it. If you just want the taste, you can try this wonderful trick I learned from a French fashion designer Justine Leconte. She recommends taking three total bites. The first she refers to as "bonjour" to welcome the experience and get a sense of the flavors and mouthfeel. The second is designed to savor and fully experience the treat. The third and final bite is "au revoir" to seal the experience and feel complete so you can move back to your tea or coffee.

■ ***Still Adhere to "Water First."*** If you're going to have something with no protein or purpose that's purely for pleasure, that's fine. I do it too sometimes, but only when I know I'm in control. And that starts with making sure I have my Water First.

■ ***Go on the Scale the Next Day.*** You may be surprised. It might not go up at all. It may even go down, because you did a lot of other things that day that were so helpful. And if it does go up, you're going to learn from it. If you avoid it, you can set yourself up for days of dissatisfaction. No need for that.

2B MINDSET SUCCESS STORY

Karla W., 36, New York, New York, lost 49 pounds in 12 months*

"I could barely get out of bed, and now I am trekking mountains!"

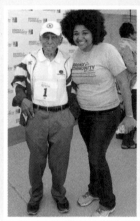 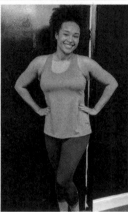

*Results vary depending on starting point and effort.

WEIGHT GAIN CAN result in an emotional bottom for many people, and that was the case with Karla W. She wasn't always overweight, but a long, dark period of her life had manifested itself in extremely unhealthy habits, and as a result her health began to suffer. It was the lowest point she had ever been—both mentally and physically. "It seemed like no matter what I tried, I was never going to be healthy again," she says. "And I was in desperate need of someone to help me figure out how to help myself."

She began 2B Mindset after the surprising end of a long-term relationship, and found journaling, while challenging to incorporate into her daily activities and busy career as a lawyer, to be especially helpful. "It taught me to be much more mindful about what I was consuming and how I was feeling," she admits. "That mindfulness was both about how I felt about what I was eating and also conscious about how I was feeling emotionally. I was able to link my emotions to my consumption much more closely." This helped her in quickly adjusting her habits—in all areas of her life.

Like many others who have given the program a chance, Karla has found that its benefits far exceed weight loss. "The 2B Mindset has helped me feel more confident and stable, understand my challenges and identify obstacles to my success more quickly, and realize that I have the capacity for great change and that the change I seek is sustainable," she says.

But most important, it helped her feel proud of herself and of her accomplishments. For the first time in her life, she suggests physical activities to her friends as social outings. Recently, she trekked down a mountain for five kilometers—over and under logs and through rivers! "I have never been more terrified and more proud of myself!" she exclaims.

CHAPTER SUMMARY

■ *The root cause of self-sabotage can be overthinking and feeling, which often drives our actions.*

■ *If you know that you frequently sabotage yourself, then counter it with clear reasoning, meaning and logical thinking.*

■ *To steel yourself against self-sabotage, set a date for your weight loss, make a realistic plan, politely pass on foods you don't need by saying, "No thanks, I'm good," and be accountable—either in your journal or to a friend.*

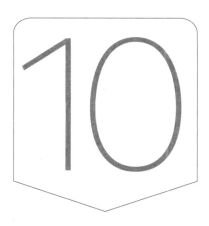

EXERCISE IS EXTRA CREDIT

Turbocharge Your Physical—
and Mental—Health
by Moving Your Body.

WHEN YOU'RE IN school, you know there are things that you have to do if you want success— completing the mandatory assignments, whether it's tests, papers or projects. You do the work, you earn the grade, you finish successfully.

And sometimes—if a teacher is especially generous—you can earn some extra credit. Remember how excited you got when you knew you had some opportunities to push your grades up a few points? It was a chance to give yourself a bump to help improve on what you have already done. Bonus time.

But it wasn't a substitute for doing the actual, real work in the class. It was exactly as the name implied: *extra*.

For a long time, exercise has been framed as one of the mandatory assignments in a weight-loss curriculum. The message seems to be: You have to sweat, sweat, sweat if you want to lose, lose, lose.

You actually see it all the time in our abs-loving, booty-flaunting Instagram culture. You gotta #grind. Sun's out, buns out! CrossFit, splat points, mud runs. The exercise culture and #fitfam is strong— and it can be fun and healthy and awesome.

In fact, it *is* fun and healthy and awesome.

But you do not have to work out around the clock to achieve the body you want.

Instead, the best way to think about exercise is as that wonderful offer of extra credit—a way to give yourself a jolt but not as a substitute for your baseline assignments. You can use exercise for what it is—an amazing opportunity to sweat out stress, clear your mind, improve your shape, feel more confident, boost your health, and ultimately, serve as an igniter of motivation that will help keep your nutrition on track.

I have always found exercise has helped me drink more water and feel more capable and energetic. However, I never saw it tick the needle on the scale unless I was making the right choices with my fork. When I came to this realization, it actually made me enjoy exercise more. I stopped exercising as an excuse to eat more "because I earned it" or "because I will burn it off later." I started to exercise to spend time with friends, learn new dance and cardio moves, listen to fun music, clear my mind and feel prouder of my body.

I want you to learn to love what exercise can do for you—and not think of it as another chore that needs to be completed every day. (As a student you never viewed extra credit as a chore, but rather as a chance.) Sometimes, thinking about changing your food habits and

2B MINDSET SUCCESS STORY

Amanda L., an Independent Team Beachbody Coach, 45, Nauvoo, Alabama,
lost 75 pounds in 19 months*

"It is a lifestyle I will follow for the rest of my life!"

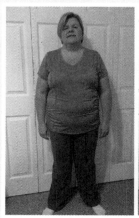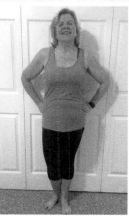

*Results vary depending on starting point and effort and following Beachbody fitness programs.

MANY IN THE 2B Mindset community have spent decades trying out different diets and trendy weight-loss program to no avail. While those diets might teach you how to count calories and weigh your food, they offer little when it comes to actually educating you about health and wellness, so that you can really understand what is going on with your body. Amanda L. tried out every diet under the sun before she found me—and 2B Mindset truly helped her become the best version of herself. "If it wasn't for the educational nutritional knowledge I have gained through your teaching, I would not be where I am now," she says. It was not only the program that helped her drop 75 pounds, but the support of the 2B social media community. "It really helped me stay consistent with the program," she says. After two months, she invested even more in herself by joining Beachbody On Demand and utilizing the daily workouts. "When I click on BOD and see I have done nearly 400 workouts since my original purchase in May of 2018, I know I am getting my money's worth," she says.

exercise habits at the same time can be too steep a mountain to climb. In order to have the most success, you have to first embrace your Core Four and make new habits when it comes to water, veggies, protein, FFCs and accessories.

The last thing I want you to sweat about is your sweat.

So let's explore the essentials of exercise—and how you can use exercise to boost your body in the best ways possible when you're ready for it.

THE EXCELLENCE OF EXERCISE

WE HAVE HAD dozens of people lose incredible amounts of weight with the 2B Mindset doing no exercise at all. In fact, many people said that the 2B Mindset was their gateway to fitness. Because it's not mandatory, people often yearn for it once they hit milestones with their weight loss. Your journey may find you focusing wholeheartedly on the 2B Mindset program to improve your weight and overall health. Eventually, hopefully when you are feeling up to it, you will *want* to work out!

Even though it's extra credit, it is worth taking some time to celebrate the benefits of exercise. These are some of my favorites.

- *It's fun!* Maybe the idea of moving your body doesn't seem very fun right now. That's fine. That feeling will subside with ongoing weight loss. Or perhaps you just can't recall ever doing exercise that felt fun, which means you need to keep exploring.

    I can tell you from personal experience that exercise is a lot more fun when you're down some pounds. I dreaded seeing my jiggle-jaggle during jumping jacks. It got in the way during crunches. And it made me feel like I was holding the world up on a plank. You might also have a memory of exercise that's dreadful because you had an instructor who made a snarky remark, you endured an injury or you didn't feel as coordinated as the regulars. But that all can change if you embrace it with an open mind and keep searching. Depending on when you choose to start, you will see that exercise can be a source of infinite fun and enjoyment in your life, especially as you keep progressing and exploring new forms.

Our bodies were designed to move. There's something for everyone to love out there. If lifting weights doesn't excite you, dance! When the music is going and you're focused on the beat, it won't feel like a workout at all. If dancing doesn't fire you up enough, box! Boxing channels your stress in such a fun and empowering way. If boxing doesn't ignite your interest, embrace the natural and super-beneficial movements of yoga and barre—these are all types of workouts that are available on Beachbody On Demand. You can do them from the comfort of your home and not worry about snide instructors or side-eye from I-take-this-class-seven-times-a-week-Susan (or anyone else). And if all else fails, just get up and take a long walk. It's one of the most basic human skills! My son started walking far before he started speaking. It's not just good for your body, it's good for your soul. It makes you feel more whole and alive. It's okay if you want to focus on your nutrition and weight loss first, but please believe that one day you will stumble on a workout that you will actually enjoy and look forward to doing.

▪ *You'll burn calories and fat.* If you remember when I talked about metabolism and fat storage, you recall that it was all about energy. The body uses your food as fuel to power systems in your body. Whatever fuel isn't used up can get stored as fat. When you're exercising, you're using up calories in order to power your body, muscles and systems, which are working harder than usual to keep you moving. In a simplified look at the caloric equation, exercise burns up energy that could otherwise get stored as fat (or uses energy from your existing body fat, allowing you to burn it off). The one caution I have is the one I mentioned earlier: Don't get lulled into thinking that you're burning a lot. Even a rigorous 45-minute workout won't burn all that much when you compare it with the total number of calories you can consume in a third of that time.

■ *It could improve your lean muscle mass.* Depending on what exercise you do, you can also increase some lean muscle mass—which can help improve your shape and help with additional calorie burn. That's because muscle is what we would call "metabolically expensive," in that it takes more calories to "feed" your muscles than it does to maintain fat, so you burn more calories when you add a little muscle.

Increased caloric burn doesn't just happen during a workout but also for the minutes following many workouts, due to the continuous twitching of muscle fibers. (So it's good if you feel the shake during that plank or squat hold!)

■ *It improves your overall wellness and health.* Research shows that exercise benefits just about every system in your body, from your skeletal system to your cardiovascular system. So as we think about obesity as a total-body health issue, it's good to also consider the numerous benefits that exercise can have on all of your systems.

■ *It can boost your mood and energy.* A lot of research links exercise to a lower risk of depression. It has been shown to improve mood, increase energy and decrease stress. That's so good for your health in and of itself, of course (who doesn't like to feel better?). But think about the effect that it has on your approach to eating. If you feel better, are less stressed and have more mental stamina, you're in a better place to shift your mindset, make good decisions and not fall prey to temptation. This comes from the endorphins produced during exercise, as well as activity's ability to help you reduce stress.

The irony of exercise is that it's easy to think that you don't have enough energy to work out when, in fact, working out gives you more energy. So while drinking more water, eating more veggies and losing weight can prop up your energy, so can regular exercise. When you consider that your mood will likely improve as you start to lose weight, this extra credit that comes from exercise makes it even more likely you're going to feel better!

I also recommend working out in front of a mirror. It might not be possible for the entirety of the workout, but working out in a place where you can see your reflection can be very powerful. While it's great to run outside or on a treadmill while watching TV, there's nothing quite like working out near a mirror and catching the reflection of your body changing. It can improve your sense of body positivity in a very impactful way. Some days the scale may stay stagnant and your motivation may ebb, but when you see definition creep into your biceps, or notice your collar bones becoming more prominent or see that your thighs are narrower, it can be massively encouraging. It's also beneficial for making sure you are maintaining proper form—which can help reduce injury.

Don't underestimate the power of this cycle: When you feel better, you eat better. When you eat better, you feel better. And you keep reaping the benefits from both. The body feeds the mind, and the mind feeds the body. As Elle Woods (Reese Witherspoon) said in *Legally Blonde*: "Exercise gives you endorphins; endorphins make you happy!"

- *It can help you sleep better.* This is important because lack of quality sleep is associated with so many health problems, but also because when you're tired and sluggish, you increase your chance of reaching for a quick "silly" carb for a boost. That starts the cascade of blood sugar spikes and drops associated with weight gain.

- *It will keep you on track as a bonus craving crusher.* If you know you have to show up to an early workout in the morning, exercise really helps you second-guess that cocktail the night before. There is a great motivational quote: "You will never always be motivated, so you must learn to be disciplined." Being on a regular fitness regimen keeps you disciplined and on your game when you might otherwise not be. This is especially true if you're held accountable by a fitness partner, Team Beachbody Coach or challenge group. Regular exercise also encourages you to incorporate other healthy habits into your life that support and enhance your workouts, like stretching, sleeping earlier and drinking more water.

- *It's another way to measure progress.* You already know how I feel about tracking—it's one of the keys to using data to inform your choices so you can see what works and what doesn't. The same is true for exercise. It's a great way to show how you're doing—whether it's improving the amount of weight you can lift or the number of minutes you can run or swim, you're able to see tangibly what happens when you get fitter. As long as you remember to take it slowly (if you're new to exercise) and not think you have to do too much out of the gate, you can track your activity and see its effect on the scale. But please manage these expectations: Just because you go all out a time or two, you're not going to see the scale plummet five pounds. The incremental weight loss will be just that—incremental.

■ ***It's a source of strength.*** I know you're going to do amazing things when you adopt the 2B Mindset and rethink your food and the way you feel day in and day out. When you see the scale move in the direction you want, you will have such a sense of power and accomplishment. You can derive even more of that when you see what you can do physically. Doing a push-up or completing a Beachbody program makes you realize that you're so much stronger than you think. It's incredibly uplifting and empowering. It can make you feel stronger in so many other areas of your life as well. As long as you remember that you don't have to climb Everest with every workout (unless you want to!), you will see exercise as a source of inner strength—to show you what you can do and what you can accomplish. And that will help propel you through every day.

And right now, how about you hold a plank? I know, I'm totally nuts, but why not? Are you in bed? That's okay— it'll only take a minute, and you probably needed to get up to pee anyway. Are you on a train, plane or in a crowded public space? Set it in your calendar to do it before the day is over. But if that's not the case, let's do this! We're all in this together!

We'll start with a kneeling plank. If you're concerned about your knees, you can lay out a folded towel underneath them. Set up your timer for 60 seconds. Start in an all-fours or tabletop position. Walk your hands forward about six inches and bring your shoulders over

8 Ways to Ease into Exercise

If you want to get started, but you're not ready to give it 100 percent, I do have some ideas for how you can ease into some easy-does-it movements just to get your body used to it—to whet your appetite, so to speak. Some ways you can sneak in some low-maintenance activity so that it doesn't feel like a burden:

- *Go for a ten-minute walk every night after dinner.*

- *While you're waiting for your morning shower to warm up, do ten standing push-ups against the bathroom wall.*

- *Every time you track exercise and don't have a workout to fill in, do 20 jumping jacks or squats.*

- *Get or build a standing desk. It encourages you to move and stretch a bit more. I absolutely love mine.*

- *Learn yoga's sun salutation and try to do it every time before you turn on your nighttime show.*

- *Make a commitment to walk along a nature trail or path once a week for at least 30 minutes. Call on a partner to join you. Get a playlist or audio book as a backup to ensure you still go if your partner cancels.*

- *When you feel stressed, set a timer for one minute and "shadow box." That's just punching air, but it can help you get your aggression out.*

your wrists. It should create a straight slope from your head to your knees at a 45-degree angle from the ground. Keep your abs engaged by pulling your belly button in and up like you're trying to squeeze into tight jeans. You got it! Start the timer!

To advance the pose, lift your knees off the floor so you are in a full push-up position. Relax the shoulders and push the ground away. Keep your abs and tush tight and right. Make it through the minute by repeating over and over "I'm okay" and "I can do this."

If you have wrist sensitivity, you can also do this on your forearms. WAY TO GO, ROCKSTAR!

You can handle anything!

THE EXPECTATIONS FOR EXERCISE

HERE'S THE MAIN reason you should think of exercise as extra credit: You should manage your expectations about its role in your overall approach to wellness and weight loss. There are many great reasons exercise is heralded as one of the best weapons in the fight for wellness, but what has happened is that we have not thought about exercise in its true context—and perhaps that has made us have unrealistic expectations about what it can do. So let's take a look at some of them:

UNREALISTIC EXPECTATION: *You Need to Work Out to Have a Weight Loss Day.*

While it may be true that everyone has the potential to move in some way, there are times when, temporarily, you just can't.

I see it in myself and with my clients. People with serious injuries, new moms post childbirth and people who have recently had surgery, for example. Or maybe something is happening at work and your schedule is jam-packed. Or maybe you are going through some major family stress and carving out time to work out just doesn't seem possible. Or your body is in need of a recovery day. The list goes on. Those aren't meant to be excuses (you'll see my approaches for excuse-proofing in Chapter 9). But they are meant to tell you that it's okay to not have to worry about exercise as you address your issues. Whenever I have someone come in with reasons they can't exercise, I don't scold them. I say, "Okay, I get it, let's focus on the food and what we can control." For many people, trying to make new habits with both food and exercise is just too much. So give yourself a break and realize that even if you can, maybe you shouldn't—at least for now.

When you get eating into a good place (and start to develop a healthier relationship with food), you'll be in a much better spot to begin with a consistent exercise program and sustain a positive relationship with your body and the food you put into it.

But as a general guideline, if two or three months go by and you're still not moving at all, you might be getting into excuse territory, so check in with yourself, your schedule and your body to see where you can fit it in.

UNREALISTIC EXPECTATION: *You Use Exercise to "Burn Off" Dessert.* I totally get it. When someone starts a program, they get super excited and want to do everything well. So you jump into a new class that your friend raves about. You try it, you like it, and wow, that was hard. So no doubt you probably burned thousands of calories! Wow, that muffin, pizza or sub looks fab! The truth is, no matter how hard you worked or how many new muscle groups you discovered because you had no idea *that* part of your body could get sore, you can't out-train bad eating. But in our minds, we justify the "cheat eat" if we had a difficult workout because we feel it was earned. That psychological trick we play on ourselves never works—and it always backfires, because you can literally negate any calorie burn you had in a workout with just a few bites.

This is truly one of the major causes of our obesity epidemic, so please don't think you're alone. If you were like me and exercising for a long time and not slimming down, you were likely underestimating how much you were eating and overestimating how much you were burning.

People think they can eat more if they exercise, and that's a negative mindset you have to get rid of.

When you put exercise in proper context—as a supplement to good nutrition, not a *substitute* for good nutrition—then you'll have much more success.

If you think this is relevant to you, I recommend taking three consecutive days off your workout plan and replace it with extra sleep, stretching or light walking. Track really well, drink plenty of water, make your meals Veggies Most and see how your appetite and scale respond. Once you see what a constructive weight-loss day looks like in terms of food, you can try incorporating the workouts as you stay consistent with the eating. Remember to always add additional water with workouts (about another 2B Mindset water bottle or 30 ounces for every 60 minutes of exercise). If you are feeling extra hungry, of course you can use the More? Sure! Model and add in a smart supplement like Beachbody Performance Recover as your protein, but be mindful of the extras beyond your typical weight-loss day.

UNREALISTIC EXPECTATION: ***You Can Just Do It if You Tough It Out!***
I've had to lose 100 pounds. You know how good it feels to be flapping around, bouncing, chafing and hurting when you're trying to move with any kind of rigor when you're *that* overweight? It feels like a cheese grater on your thighs, it feels like you're carrying a fridge on your back, and it feels like you're huffing and puffing with hurricane-force winds.

It. Hurts.

And no amount of "toughness" can change the fact that your thigh skin feels like rug burn. But what happens when we try to go really hard at the start of a program and realize that we can't push it like our minds want us to? We feel like we failed. We feel like it's a lost cause. And we feel that instead of curling weights, we might as well curl a dozen mini doughnuts to our mouth.

So in your mind, you have to change the narrative about what you can do right from the start—and you have to manage what you want to do versus what you can do. Use modifiers as needed and start at a level that feels right for you but leaves room for growth. It's important to realize that exercise sometimes gets harder before it gets easier. There may be soreness and new coordination to get used to in the beginning, but it does get easier with practice, improved muscle memory, preparation and recovery methods, and comfortability. Plus of course as you lose weight—through proper nutrition—your body will start to feel better, and you'll be able to do more and more. And that's when you'll really reap the benefits of exercise.

It's okay to find something that suits your current abilities, which may start with walking around the block once a day. It all counts, and you'll be doing laps around everyone sitting on the couch. You are also creating the foundations of a good habit so be proud of any and all your extra credit!

UNREALISTIC EXPECTATION: *You Can Handle It All.*

It takes a lot of spirit and motivation to do what you're doing right now—committing to a new way of eating, a new way of life and a new body, too. And I know you're ready to make changes, but to think you can just snap your fingers and change eating and exercise habits at the same time is a *lot* to handle. Part of your challenge—in the short term— is pulling the reins on your excitement and knowing that it's okay to take your time. It's not a matter of whether you can handle a shift in eating and exercise for a week or two; it's a matter of dealing with it over the long haul. And your best chance for success comes from taking it one change at a time. As I just said, maybe the exercise component starts with something as basic as walking around the block or doing those push-ups against the bathroom wall. You are doing wonders for your health by taking on the 2B Mindset; this is meant to feel uplifting, that's why it's called extra credit!

UNREALISTIC EXPECTATION: *Exercise Is an Instant Fat Melter.*

It's true—exercise burns calories, builds muscle and changes your shape. But exercise is not a time machine. You can't step into a spin class for a week or two and expect to see grand results. This can be deflating for lots of people—especially my husband, who expects to look like Thor after 30 minutes of weightlifting. After all, if you start to work out an hour a day, shouldn't you be a size smaller in two weeks? Uh, no. And that's where it can be demoralizing. You feel like you should be making faster gains when you've engaged in a new routine. So part of it is about being patient—and realizing that you can't do it all.

When you keep your expectations in check, that's when you can really benefit from all of the good things that can happen when you do start a new exercise routine.

So what should you expect from exercise? That it has the potential—when you're ready—to be a constant source of happiness, strength and stress relief and keep your mindset focused, positive and strong.

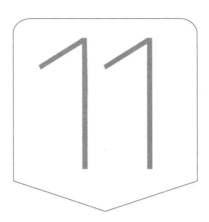

MAINTENANCE MODE

Stick to Your Goal Weight,
and Never Look Back.

KEEP FOLLOWING 2B Mindset and you should never gain back your weight. My clients don't gain it back! Many people in the first-ever 2B Mindset test group also kept it off! I know this sounds like science fiction or too good to be true, but if you follow the plan, a day will come when you don't want to drop weight anymore. You won't have any more to drop! You'll no longer be in Weight Loss Mode or Melting Mode. You'll be in Maintenance Mode, and in this chapter, we'll go over what that looks like.

Eating and Drinking in Maintenance Mode

If you've reached your goal weight, I recommend continuing 2B Mindset as you've been doing it—Water First, Veggies Most, Track It, Use the Scale. Then you can play with what modifications you'll need. If you lose more weight, you'll figure out pretty shortly how you can change things. For example:

- **You might add more food.** You might want to make your dinner plate look more like your lunch plate—or add an extra snack. Or you may have room for more FFCs or silly treats. The goal is to figure out what maintaining looks like while still developing that positive relationship with food. There's a trial and error to it.

- **You might play with your schedule.** Some people maintain their weight best by eating very similarly Monday to Friday because those are the recipes and meal patterns they're used to. In which case, maybe there's extra room to relax and enjoy a few extra treats on the weekends. That way, Monday to Friday you might see a pound go off, and then Friday to Sunday you might see a pound come on. Overall you're maintaining your weight.

- **You might adapt depending on your workouts.** Let's say you've started a really rigorous regimen and want to add in a post-workout protein shake, like Beachbody Performance Recover, to maintain your weight while building muscle. Go for it.

Tracking in Maintenance Mode

In the first few weeks of Maintenance Mode, your tracking should be as detailed as possible.

- **Track everything.** How many hours are you sleeping? How many water ounces are you drinking? What times are you eating? Continue to ask yourself why you're eating: Is it physical hunger? Is it emotional? Is it habit hunger? Is it sense hunger, because it's just in front of your face?

- **Add your feelings.** This only gives you greater awareness. Sometimes I'll jot down: *"I ate my daughter's cookies."* Or I'll be more detailed than that: *"I ate three of my daughter's cookies. Totally unnecessary, not even worth it."* The more you put in, the more you can learn. Even today, I do this all the time. If I'm eating and I'm super stressed, I write it down. I also love to put down things I'm happy about. I'll write: *"I had two cock-tails. I had some of my husband's fries and I really enjoyed them."*

- **Remain in touch with what leads to weight gain.** With those added notations in the tracker, I then don't care when the scale goes up—it's fine. I now understand that those kinds of treats mean half a pound of change and not a three-pound change. I have also learned that if I had stopped at the two cocktails—if I didn't have the fries—maybe I would have maintained my weight. The more details you put into the tracker, the more you get out of it.

Using the Scale in Maintenance Mode

Keep in touch with the scale every day. If I have a client who hits their goal weight, I'll ask, "What are you going to do with the scale?" If they say, "Well, I'm in the habit of using it every day, so I'm probably just going to continue that," I'll say, "Toodle-loo!" I'll never have to see them again because they know exactly what to do, but I will see their friends, cousins or uncles trying to book an appointment with me.

- **Expect a balance.** Maintenance is kind of like a balancing game—you won't stay at the exact same weight. Expect about a five-pound range. If you start at the bottom of the range, you might go to the top of the range after a vacation. But you know exactly how to go back into weight loss mode: go back to the two bunnies, especially your tracker; go back to everything you need to do, and reflect on those great weight-loss days. Bring them back, and get back into a comfortable spot where you feel happy and confident.

- **Manage your expectations.** When weighing in, you may feel let down. I know that sounds perverse because you've already reached your goal weight—what's to feel bad about!?! But because you won't be witnessing progress every day—seeing the scale go down, down, down—or working toward a goal, it may be a bummer. Find another goal or hobby while you maintain your weight, like implementing a fitness program or finishing a book series.

2B MINDSET SUCCESS STORY

Susan M., 43, Lawrence, Georgia, lost 60 pounds in 7 months*

"It's not only the scale victories that have me so excited!"

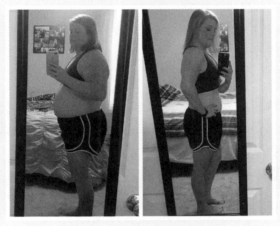

*Results vary depending on starting point and effort.

A LOT OF PEOPLE who start the 2B Mindset program focus on the numbers on the scale. They are pleasantly surprised to learn that there are so many other ways their lives and bodies transform as a result of weight loss. Susan M. was one of the many people who have reaped endless lifestyle and health benefits due to 2B Mindset. "It's not only the scale victories that have me so excited," she exclaims. "Other than being sixty pounds lighter and three sizes smaller in clothes, I have a ton of energy." Additionally, her ring and watch sizes have gone down significantly. But the best surprise of all was the simplicity of the program. "My mindset changed when I saw how easy the program was to follow, and it just clicked and became my new way of thinking," she says. Of all the things I taught her, the one that resonates the most with Susan is the concept of "simple, sensible, sustainable." "The 2B Mindset program is all that for me and why I know I will never go back to the old, overweight person I used to be. It's the best thing you can do for you!"

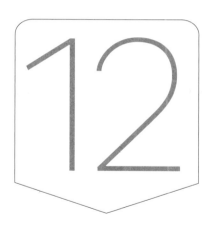

LET'S KEEP DOING THIS TOGETHER— ONLINE!

Lock in Your Weight Loss by Signing Up for 2B Mindset and The Mindset Membership.

YOU WILL LOSE weight by applying everything you've learned in this book. But I don't just want you to lose weight. I want you to be able to keep it off for good! And that's why I encourage you to do something for yourself that you deserve. Sign up for 2B Mindset and the Mindset Membership.

I've put it all out there for you at try2Bmindset.com. You'll have the equivalent of thousands of dollars in private counseling with me. It's like having regular sessions with me in my private practice! I know my private sessions aren't accessible to everyone; that's why I've created the 2B Mindset and The Mindset Membership—a companion program to 2B Mindset that gives you ongoing support in so many ways. But the best part? The program and a year of the membership cost less than one private session with me!

Along with this book, you'll have every tool you need to lose weight happily and keep it off for good. The 2B Mindset is a digital video-based program, broken up into more than 40 short segments that you can watch anywhere on any device. While this book talks you through many of the principles, the videos provide a deeper understanding. You'll see firsthand how the 2B Mindset translates successfully into practice and your life—I am sharing more of my favorite tips and secrets. The videos are fun and easy to watch. They'll help you keep learning and having success as you create more new healthy habits. In addition to doing a deeper dive with the program's fundamentals, I also teach you how to set up your kitchen for success and so much more.

One of the coolest things about 2B Mindset is its seamless integration into your everyday life. You're already going to the grocery store; in the Grocery Store Tour video, I'll be right there with you, showing you how to do it so you can reach your goals, plus save money at checkout and save time in the kitchen.

If you love to cook or are just getting started with spending more time in the kitchen, you're going to love the recipe videos! I'll show you how to make delicious, yummy recipes that are super simple with minimal ingredients. If you've never cooked before in your life—as in, you don't remember how to turn on your oven—you'll love to watch. I certainly don't come from a culinary background, and I think that the fewer ingredients required and the easier to make, the better the recipe. So by default, these are simple-to-make, yummy, big, filling, satisfying meals. If you are more of a gourmet, you'll still love to watch my slim-down techniques and apply them to your favorite creations.

Don't want to cook at all? Totally fine. In the Enjoy Takeout Food video, I'll show you how to order Thai, Japanese, Chinese, Italian and many other cuisines the 2B Mindset way, so you can still eat all these delicious foods and cuisines you enjoy and keep losing weight.

You'll also find videos about issues that might have tripped you up in the past, including how to handle travel and vacations (with specifics for a business trip, weekend getaway or a longer vacation), and how to go to events like Thanksgiving dinner or football Sundays. I also talk about cocktail parties, weddings—every kind of event.

No matter what question, hurdle or struggle you've hit along the way in your weight-loss and fitness journey, this is an effective support system for it. I walk you through every step of the way so you can get to the weight you want to be.

Here are all the tools you'll get either online or delivered to your door when you get the comprehensive 2B Mindset program.

The Videos

As I mentioned earlier, I created a series of videos in which I teach you the program, step by step. Each video is like a one-on-one private session with me. Watch the videos by logging in to 2BMindset.com or the app (more on that below) so you can tap into the 2B Mindset whenever or wherever. Any time you're in a rut, watch or rewatch a video. (You will be extra-thankful for Start Losing Weight Now; Make Over Your Mindset; and Help! I'm at a Plateau!)

My Tracker

One convenient place to track each day's weight, water and food intake, plus helpful planning pages that make it simple to fit the 2B Mindset into your daily life! You may not think that tracking is for you, but doing it is imperative to reach your weight-loss goals. It takes just a few minutes each day—and I promise it will be well worth your time!

You may think that any ordinary notepad or phone app could work, but I designed this tracker based on my experience with hundreds of clients, removing the waste that you may see in other food trackers and including everything you need to fully adopt the mindset, lose weight and keep it off. You'll learn what a "weight-loss day" looks like so you can keep your mindset—and your weight loss—on track. You can track in the book, with the interactive PDF and also in the app.

Extended Content

The digital database is packed with more of my exclusive recipes, flexible meal plans, with easy-to-follow shopping lists, season-specific recipes, a kitchen and pantry guide, ways to mix and match my favorite foods, dining-out guides and so much more.

Water Bottle

I hope if you're this far into the book you're already saying "Water First!" just like I do. As you know by now, I want you to drink lots of water throughout the day! That's why I've included an exclusive 2B Mindset water bottle, with motivational reminders to keep you on track all day. I specifically designed this water bottle to include features that will get you drinking water—and loving it! People tell me it's one of their favorite parts of the program and have even gifted the bottles to friends and family.

The App

This is your go-to place to access the entire 2B Mindset program:
- *Watch the videos.*
- *Preview the downloadable and printable tools and resources.*
- *Track your water, weight, Shakeology and daily food intake, even take pictures of your plate for ease.*

■ *Quickly access the recipes and meal plans so you can refer to them in the market if you forgot to plan ahead.*

■ *To download, go to the app store on your mobile phone and search for "Beachbody."*

Your Own Personal Coach and Community Support

I will definitely give you ongoing support when you sign up for The Mindset Membership, but I can only help you so much with your individual quirks and questions. Your Coach will be the one who will be with you every day and every step of the way. Once you sign up for 2B Mindset you can contact your Coach through the My Account section of TeamBeachbody.com.

When you join The Mindset Membership, you'll get access to:

■ *A Monthly Topic Video:* We kick off each month with a topic requested by the community. Every topic focuses on relatable, real-life experiences for which I provide insights and strategies on how to overcome obstacles and stay focused on your goals, such as Following the Plan on a Budget and More Strategies to Crush Late-Night Cravings. In every video I will be joined by a few lucky Mindset members (which could one day be you!).

■ *A Goal-Setting Worksheet:* During the Monthly Topic video, you'll have the opportunity to fill out a corresponding worksheet designed to keep you accountable by setting goals for the month and identifying helpful habits to implement so you can stay on track.

■ *A One-on-One Video:* Each month, one lucky Mindset member will get the opportunity to have a one-on-one session with me. During this video session, I will get to know that member's lifestyle, habits and goals and review their tracker so I can provide my best advice personalized for them so they can lose those next few pounds. These intimate, powerful one-on-one conversations are eye-opening and help you fully understand all the factors in someone's day-to-day journey. And the best part? The next selected member could be you!

- *A Tracker Takeaway Worksheet:* I'll provide a "Tracker Takeaway" worksheet for you, so you can take notes as you learn new ways to track as you watch the One-on-One video.

- *Monthly Meal Plans:* Each month I will feature a brand new seven-day meal plan based on 2B Mindset recipes to help make it even easier to stay on track and reach your goals. Whether you follow the regular or vegan plan, there's an option that fits your lifestyle.

- *LIVE Office Hours:* To help everyone stay connected to their goals and get their questions answered, I will host live Office Hours each month in the Exclusive Community.

- *Exclusive Recipes:* Each week, you'll get brand-new recipes that can't be found anywhere else—for a total of eight new recipes per month. Ranging from seasonal dishes to comforting classics, each delicious recipe will come with a corresponding video and downloadable PDF so you can cook with ease and never face food fatigue.

- *Exclusive Community:* As a Mindset member you have 24/7 access to our Mindset Membership Exclusive Community. This private group is where we learn, grow and support each other on our 2B Mindset journeys. This community was created for you to post your victories, ask questions, share your thoughts and keep your habits in check. This is where you will join us for live Office Hours, and frequent check-ins from me!

Find 2B Mindset and The Mindset Membership at:

Try2bmindset.com

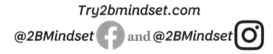

THE FINAL WORD

You Can Drop It!

BEFORE I SEND you on your way, try this last exercise for a lasting change. When you're experiencing a sense of slipping into old habits, identify them immediately and repeat the following:

This is just a craving. ■ *I can drop it.*

This is just an excuse. ■ *I can drop it.*

This is just another sugary dessert. ■ *I can drop it.*

This is self-sabotaging. ■ *I can drop it.*

This is a negative belief I tell myself. ■ *I can drop it.*

I've battled with this excess weight for far too long. ■ *I can drop it.*

I care about my future goals and what I want to be. ■ *I'm going to get it!*

ACKNOWLEDGMENTS

THE 2B MINDSET is the result of decades of thought put into how to lose weight, and *You Can Drop It!* couldn't have come together without the help of the most thoughtful team in the world. I want to thank:

God for blessing my imperfect self with this perfect life.

Noah for giving me the confidence to share my story and for bringing joy to the journey.

My kids, Olivia Rose and Julian Matan, for their curiosities and laughter that make every day better and brighter.

My grandparents and mother, Z"L, father, Emil, stepmother, in-laws, sisters, brothers, nieces, nephews and my entire family, for loving me no matter what.

My strong, smart and beautiful best friends for being my extended family and support system.

Kaitlin Blocker for being my 2B partner-in-prime and devoting her energy, time and passion to help bring this vision—and mission—to life.

Carl Daikeler, Lara Ross, Denis Faye (and his team of nutrition ninjas), Matt Tolerico, Heather Church, Garry Pay, Krista Maguire, Kirsten Morningstar, Diane Wade, Kimberly Caspari, Kate Bissegger, Mat Gonzales and my entire Beachbody family for always believing in the power of the 2B Mindset.

Michael Freidson, David Zinczenko, Joe Heroun, Laura White, Ted Spiker, Rebecca Maines and the entire team at Galvanized Media and Simon & Schuster for making this book possible—and such a gem.

And to you, the reader, for being brave enough to drop your negative self-talk, excuses and limiting beliefs and bring this positive mindset into your life. I'm truly so thankful and excited for you.

INDEX

D